Occupational Stress

PERSONAL AND PROFESSIONAL APPROACHES

Edited by

Sally Hardy
Lecturer
School of Health, Department of Nursing and Midwifery, University of East Anglia

Jerome Carson
Senior Lecturer in Clinical Psychology
Institute of Psychiatry, London

and

Honorary Consultant Clinical Psychologist
The Bethlem and Maudsley NHS trust, London

and

Ben Thomas
Chief Nursing Advisor
The Maudsley Hospital, London

Stanley Thornes (Publishers) Ltd

First published in 1998 by:
Stanley Thornes (Publishers) Ltd
Ellenborough House
Wellington Street
CHELTENHAM
GL50 1YW
United Kingdom

98 99 00 01 / 10 9 8 7 6 5 4 3 2 1

A catalogue record for this book is available from the British Library

ISBN 0-7487-3302-7

Typeset by Columns Design Ltd, Reading
Printed and bound in Great Britain
by T.J. International, Padstow, Cornwall

Occupational Stress

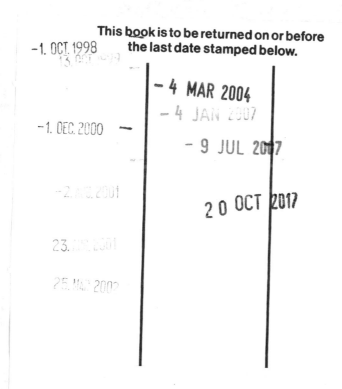

Contents

Contributors

Catherine Adcock
Clinical Charge Nurse, The Bethlem Royal Hospital, Monks Orchard Road, Beckenham, Kent BR3 3BX

Sydney Brandon
Emeritus Professor of Psychiatry, University of Leicester; Chairman, National Counselling Service for Sick Doctors

Tony Butterworth
Professor and Dean of School of Nursing, Midwifery and Health Visiting, University of Manchester, Oxford Road, Manchester M13 9PL

Jerome Carson
Senior Lecturer in Clinical Psychology, Institute of Psychiatry, Denmark Hill, London SE5 8AF

Cary L. Cooper
Professor of Organizational Psychology, Manchester School of Management, UMIST, PO Box 88, Manchester M60 1QD

Mike Gill
Senior Lecturer, Department of Psychiatry, Trinity Centre for Health Sciences, St James' Hospital, James' Street, Dublin 8, Republic of Ireland

Vedan Gunnoo
Senior Lecturer Mental Health, South Bank University, London SE1 0AA

Sally Hardy
Lecturer, School of Health, University of East Anglia, Management Centre, Hellesdon Hospital, Norwich NR6 5BE

Patrick Hopkinson
Clinical Service Manager, Southside Partnership, Scout Lane, Clapham, London
SW4 0LA

Elizabeth Kuipers
Reader in Clinical Psychology, Institute of Psychiatry, Denmark Hill, London SE5
8AF

Jan Long
Staff Support Service Manager, 7 The Mall, Swindon, Wiltshire SN1 4JA

Kathleen A. Moore
Senior Lecturer in Clinical Psychology, School of Psychology, Deakin University,
Burwood, Victoria, Australia

Christopher Rance
Senior Management Consultant and Group Analyst, Rance Management Systems
Ltd, 43 Rosendale Road, London SE21 8DY

David Sines
Professor of Community Nursing/Head of School of Health Sciences,
Newtownabbey, Co. Antrim, Northern Ireland BT37 0QB

Mark Sutherland
Chaplain, The Maudsley Hospital, Denmark Hill, London SE5 8AZ

Ben Thomas
Chief Nursing Advisor, Administration Building, The Maudsley Hospital,
Denmark Hill, London SE5 8AZ

P. Joe Tobin
Psychologist, South Eastern Health Board, Community Care Headquarters,
James' Green, Kilkenny, Republic of Ireland

Foreword

It is not enough for us to do what we can do;
the patient and his environment, and external
conditions have to achieve the cure.

Hippocrates 460–370 BC

While conducting studies on the causes of stress the physiologist Cannon commented that '… the temptation is strong to suggest that some phases of those pathological states [in stress] are associated with the strenuous and exciting character of modern life …'. Today, nearly a century later, we have progressed little in taking this understanding forward in a way that is helpful to those suffering stress; we merely pick up the pieces and stumble on – a far cry from the understanding demonstrated by Hippocrates that the environment and external conditions are important to the individual and their carers. There are many reasons why this excellent publication is timely, indeed long overdue. While stress levels in professional carers have always been known, anecdotally if not scientifically, as being high, little has been done across the spectrum of health care to alleviate the situation. Thus the opportunity is missed to support professional carers and perhaps prevent damaging stress levels. Today, stress levels in health care staff are visibly high. 'Macho' management styles, an environment of continuous change unharnessed from any real security, and a justifiably demanding public are the only constants in most professional carers' lives. This can only be a recipe for disaster – as is often highlighted by the media – unless a framework is in place which takes account of these stressors and the needs of those providing professional care.

The authors of this well thought out book are ideally placed to take the lead on caring for professional carers. Each contributor draws on their particular knowledge and experiences in a way that places the reader in context as well as providing them with a sound academic framework within which to consider the breadth of the subject. This is a rare gift to any reader, particularly those who are less than comfortable with heavy academic style. This is not a book only for students, though as such it will be invaluable, it is a book for managers and wise commissioners of services, as it will inform the enlightened in their development of future policies to support quality care.

It is well acknowledged within the text that empowered staff are less stressed, and that support mechanisms need to be in place within the working environment to ensure that such empowerment is properly understood. Clinical supervision is such a mechanism and one which, in my view, is crucial to the success of well adjusted staff who are able to meet the demands concomitant with the provision of health and social care. The first multi-site study to evaluate the effectiveness of clinical supervision in health care settings, discussed in this text, provides an important but early step in the journey that must be taken if we are to keep our valued staff and help them to achieve professional maturity.

Burnout, one of the more obvious symptoms of stress, is not something that many admit to when I ask participants at seminars and conferences – even after I have admitted that I suffered from it myself after working for some time in an intensive care unit. Those who do, look embarrassed, as if admitting to a fault in their professional conduct. This book is a breakthrough in that it draws together the combined expertise of the authors to provide a major contribution to the body of knowledge on stress levels in professional carers. The next step must be to embed the words into our culture, and care for our invaluable but rarely cared for carers.

Professor Veronica A. Bishop
Hawkhurst, Kent, July 1997.

PART ONE

Theories of stress among mental health professionals

1

Kathleen Moore and Cary L. Cooper

Stress is universal and everyone, if asked, will tell you that they know what stress is. However, the actual usage and meaning of the word 'stress' in everyday language is highly diverse. Statements such as: 'I am under stress' (noun); 'My job is stressing me' (verb); or 'It's all too stressful' (adjective) are heard frequently. These comments are highly generalized and, at the same time, confused in terms of a universal meaning. How, as scientists and practitioners, do we address these issues? Are we any less confused as to what stress 'is'? How do we quantify people's levels of stress? It is the aim of this chapter to review the major theories of stress, their extension within an occupational context, and to examine how each of these theories contributes to the measurement of stress, with particular emphasis on one such device: the Occupational Stress Indicator.

HISTORICAL OVERVIEW

Early clinical observations dating back to the time of Galen linked personality, illness, and what we now term stress. In the first quarter of this century, physicians, such as Sir William Osler, pointed out that cancer-prone patients exhibited common characteristics such as a tendency to suppress emotions like fear and anger and an inability to react appropriately to stressful situations. Despite this wisdom, it is really only during the present century that the recognition of and the scientific investigation into the phenomenon of stress and its effects upon physical and mental well-being have burgeoned. The broad perspectives that have emerged will be described in terms of their theoretical rationale with reference to their measurement and their strengths and weakness.

STRESS AS A STIMULUS

This view includes a focus on the environment, where stress is seen as a *stimulus* – something that triggers a response – in other words, a cause. For example, statements like: 'My job is stressing me' highlight people's reference to an event or set of circumstances as the source or cause of their tension. Therefore events or cirumstances perceived as threatening or harmful, produce feelings of tension sometimes referred to as 'strain'.

Research following this stimulus approach can be divided into four broad categories: (1) catastrophic events (e.g. earthquakes), (2) major life events (e.g. loss of loved one), (3) daily hassles (e.g. missed appointments), and (4) chronic circumstances, such as living or working in crowded or noisy conditions. The stimulus theory of stress would hold that all of these events require some level of adjustment by the persons experiencing them. In this approach, stress is used to indicate the precipitating event or force applied to the individual.

Measurement of stimuli

Drawing upon their own clinical experience and supported by subsequent interview data, Holmes and Rahe (1967) developed their Social Readjustment Rating Scale (SRRS). This is probably the most widely known and adapted scale in this area; others, such as the Life Experiences Survey (LES) (Sarason, Johnson and Siegel, 1978) and the PERI Life Events Scale (Dohrenwend *et al.*, 1978), have adopted a similar methodology although with modified scoring systems.

The SRRS lists a range of major life events accompanied by a point system gauging the level of social adjustment required by that event. Respondents indicate which events they have experienced over a previous period of time, generally 12 or 24 months, and an aggregate is obtained from all items checked. Death of a spouse is rated highest at 100, whereas at the lower end, Christmas rates 12. Each person's total score is said to indicate their level of exposure to stressors which in turn, suggests each individual's attendant susceptibility to illness. Lower scores are considered healthy and, depending upon the actual range of their scores, persons scoring at higher levels may need to adjust their lifestyle to varying degrees in order to avoid potential ill health.

While the SRRS can be completed quickly and easily it is not without criticisms. Some items are vague and ambiguous; they fail to indicate 'how much' change has occurred or the 'direction' of the change; there is no distinction between desirable and undesirable events; and no account of impact for individuals based upon their personal or environmental circumstances (e.g. a £20,000 mortgage to one person may be a tremendous burden associated with high levels of worry and stress yet be of small consequence to others). Adaptations to the SRRS have attempted to deal with some of these issues although other concerns about it remain valid. For instance, Goldberg and Comstock (1980) found that the number of life events reported by people decreased with age from early adulthood to old age yet increased with the number of years of schooling. Also, single, separated, and divorced people reported a larger number of events than married and widowed individuals amongst those surveyed.

The stimulus model of stress is restricted in its generalizability, as it implies that all persons will react in similar ways to similar circumstances. This is clearly not so, as there are considerable inter-person and intra-person differences across stimuli and across time. This idiosyncratic nature of the stress response (Appley and Trumbull, 1967) has prompted researchers to view stimuli from different perspectives: (1) stress as a response of the individual, where the nature and intensity of the stressing agent are largely irrelevant, and (2) stress as the interaction of characteristics of the person and factors in the environment (Ross and Altmaier, 1994). This last also has implications for both a vulnerability model of stress and for a cybernetic model of stress (see below).

STRESS AS A RESPONSE

Cannon (1932) described stress in terms of the body's response to demands or stressors placed upon it. This response is observed in the activation of the sympathetic nervous system which, Cannon states, prepares the body to either flee from or fight the demand. Once the demand has passed, the parasympathetic nervous system returns the body to homeostasis or equilibrium.

Selye extended the response model in two major ways. Firstly, his *General Adaption Syndrome (GAS)* (Selye, 1956) describes what he calls a 'non-specific response of the body to any demand' (p. 55) placed upon it, whether external or internal, and, secondly, he attributes three phases to stress: alarm reaction, resistance, and exhaustion. Like Cannon, Selye suggests that the body is simultaneously struggling to achieve homeostasis.

During the *alarm* phase, there is a brief period of lowered resistance followed by a time of heightened arousal wherein the body prepares itself for a rapid response. Selye's response phase also involves the sympathetic nervous system: such functions as bladder and digestive activities, non-essential to immediate survival, are suspended while heart rate and the secretion of adrenaline and noradrenaline are increased together with a release of glucose, to provide the body with defences to combat the stressor.

The second stage, *resistance*, replaces the alarm phase with responses that promote long-term adaptation. The body is now prepared to challenge the stressor and continues to adapt or habituate to the stressor during this stage although this may not always be at a conscious level. The body is said to be under *strain* at this time.

The third and final stage is *collapse*. The body cannot go on resisting indefinitely. The energy for continued adjustment becomes depleted and the individual becomes exhausted. This stage marks the depletion of resources to resist; the person may then become vulnerable to tissue damage, disease, or even (as in Selye's animal studies) death.

Measurement of response/strain

Strain is the response to the stimulus and can be measured both physiologically and by pencil-and-paper reports. Increase in pulse rate, blood pressure, galvanic skin response (GSR), and muscle tension are some of the ways by which strain is measured. Other important indicators of strain include mood and anxiety questionnaires, evaluation of eating and sleeping habits, increases in negative health behaviours such as smoking and drinking, decreases in health promoting behaviours (such as exercise), and even measures of job dissatisfaction and absenteeism.

Whilst Selye has made a significant contribution to the study of stress, the GAS is in fact limited by its main premise, i.e. the proposition that the body responds in a relatively constant way regardless of the type of stimulus (stressor), and that the same response (strain) can be be elicited by pleasant or unpleasant stimuli. Certainly, Shedletsky and Endler (1974) found different physiological responses to the threat of an electric shock to those produced by the threat of rejection and disapproval by others. When applied to occupational stress, this model may account for stressors caused by certain job conditions, such as excessive noise; however, it appears inadequate to explain diverse individual reactions to complex job conditions such as role ambiguity, role conflict, or role overload.

It is important, however, to remember another of Selye's contributions to this literature, *eustress*, which ironically, is termed a stimulus. Eustress, or 'good stress', acts as a stimulus or motivator necessary to promote growth and development.

INTERACTIONAL MODELS OF STRESS

Stress has more recently and comprehensively been described as a process that includes both stressors and strains. This process involves continuous interactions and adjustments, called 'transactions', between the individual and the environment, with each affecting and being affected by the other (Cox, 1978; Lazarus and Folkman, 1984). Many of these models perceive the relationship between the individual and the environment as dynamic, with the individual influencing the impact of stress through behavioural, cognitive, and emotional strategies. Others, such as Frankenhaeuser (1993), focus more on the psychobiological mechanisms involved in job stress. This section will address some of the major person–environment models.

Holland's person–environment fit

Early person–environment fit models include Holland's (1973) concept of 'congruence' whereby individuals' vocational preference matches the arena in which they actually work. Holland proposed six vocational types: realistic, social, enterprising, investigative, artistic, and conventional. People's hierarchy of interests can be determined by a three category preference derived from a hexagonal model in which the types that are most similiar are closest together while those most dis-similar are furthest apart. For example, a profile of 'SEA' suggests that the person's predominant interest is social, followed by enterprising and artistic.

While considerable interest has focused upon this 'matching' process at both a selection level and the level of job satisfaction, there do not appear to be any data relevant to congruence and job stress. Nor has the relevance of personality vari-ables, such as sociotrophy, autonomy, and coping styles been 'matched' in rela-tion to congruence and job stress.

Psychobiological stress findings

The work of Marianne Frankenhaeuser and colleagues has dominated the arena of psychobiological stress research. While Frankenhaeuser (1993) stated that 'cogni-tive assessment of environmental demand is a key concept on our biopsychosocial approach to stress' (p. 2), much regard for her work focuses on the identification of biological markers of stress.

Relationships between blue-collar workers, repetitive work cycles, their lack of communication with fellow workers, lack of control over work pace, and verbal reports of job dissatisfaction and stress are reflected in increased catecholamine secretion (Frankenhaeuser and Gardell, 1976). Further investigations led Frankenhaeuser and colleagues to identify environmental characteristics that pro-mote either active, positive attitudes or passive, negative moods, each of these being identified with different patterns of neuroendocrine response. In brief, they report that epinephrine is a general (non-specific) indicator of intensity of arousal while increases in cortisol tend to occur only during negative affective states (Frankenhaeuser, 1991). This idea of a generalized and a specific response seems both to confirm and extend Selye's GAS model. Further research in this area is examining gender, age, and occupational differences as well as the moderating effects of social support.

Other physical manifestations of 'stress reactivity' include elevated blood pres-sure and heart rate which have also been associated with cardiovascular disease (e.g. Krantz et al., 1988). One approach to dealing with such stress reactions is to identify reactivity areas and provide training to reduce that reactivity (e.g. reduc-tions in heart rate reactivity) (Sharpley, 1994). However, Camerson (personal com-munication) says it should not be assumed that a physiological rather than a psychological solution is always the answer, and nor should it be assumed that psychological answers are insufficient. An example of this argument comes from Taylor and Frazer's (1980) finding that personnel required to recover fragmented bodies from the Mt Erebus air disaster in Antarctica were unable to eat meat for several weeks afterwards. Whilst some physiological indicators may have corre-lated with the inability to eat meat, the cognitive processes involved in confront-ing and dealing with this stressful event were clearly relevant.

Demand–discretion model of job stress

Karasek (1979) describes two orthogonal dimensions reflecting a person–environment fit: demand (quantitative workload and time pressures) and discretion (the individual's opportunity to control, participate, and engage in decision making). A perfect positive correlation, drawn through low demand / low discretion to high demand / high discretion, called the *activity* dimension, has two poles labelled 'passive' and 'active', respectively. Whilst 'active' jobs may promote greater job skills or even job satisfaction, Karasek *et al.* (1981) suggested there is no significant implication between this dimension and health.

A negative correlational axis passing through the low demand / high discretion and high demand / low discretion quadrants is termed 'strain' with the extremes labelled 'low strain' and 'high strain'. On this axis, high demand is not paralleled by similarly high levels of control or participation in decision making. Whilst some evidence has been provided for a link between this factor and cardiovascular disease (Karasek and Theorell, 1990) this model fails to address important personality and mediating variables which may hide such a relationship. Recently, Parkes, Mendham and von Rabenau (1994) partly addressed this problem. They questioned whether the impact of social support upon the demand–discretion model of job stress was additive (that is, the impacts on demand and discretion are independent) or interactive (that is, moderating between demand and discretion). Their results supported a three-way interactive model for somatic symptoms (demand $\times$ discretion $\times$ support interaction), while job satisfaction was predicted by a direct effect for support and a demand $\times$ discretion interaction.

This model has addressed the interaction amongst workload and individuals' control over that workload; subsequent investigations applying it have looked at the effect of social support. However, other factors, such as the relevance of the stimuli and any subsequent strain they induce, and the influence individuals' initial perceptions and ongoing evaluations contribute, have not been taken into account. Cognitive approaches to stress have attempted to address these issues.

COGNITIVE MODELS OF STRESS

Perhaps the most widely known of these models is the transactional model proposed by Lazarus and colleagues (Lazarus, 1966; Lazarus and Folkman, 1984). This model defines stress as occurring when there is an imbalance, or gap, between the individual's perceived demands and the perceived resources to meet those demands. It emphasizes the ongoing and dynamic nature of this 'balancing process' and suggests that individuals can influence, either in reality or perceptually, both sides of this equation, thus narrowing the gap.

Lazarus' model begins when a person evaluates a particular situation or demand, called *primary appraisal*. This perception focuses on the likelihood of negative outcomes. An appraisal of *harm* suggests that some damage has already occurred, while an appraisal of *threat* refers to harm that will most likely happen in the future should the *status quo* remain. However, appraisal is not always necessarily negative. Lazarus also refers to an *appraisal of challenge*, where individuals believe they can achieve a positive outcome, not merely protecting against a negative one.

Secondary appraisal follows; it is characterized by the individual's attempt to define what coping options are available for dealing with the harm, forestalling the threat, or to meet the challenge. These options might be resource based, may take the form of a response, be of an internal or an external nature, and they may be adaptive or maladaptive in outcome. For example, a worker experiencing difficulties might utilize the assistance or advice of others as a source of external resources, while a maladaptive form of coping would be to internalize one's 'hopelessness' and quit the job. A *sine qua non* of this model is that the perceived lack of sufficient availablility of coping resources has a strong influence in the secondary appraisal of the event or situation as stressful.

An integral component of Lazarus' model is the cognitive appraisal of life events and the resources available to deal with them. Individual variations of perception for each of these components partly address the question of inter-person and intra-person differences in relation to stress levels or the gap between demand and resources at any one time. Less clearly addressed is the impact of daily hassles in this model. Moving from a stimulus-centred view of hassles (Lazarus, 1984), Lazarus and Folkman (1984) hypothesized that 'whereas daily hassles would be normally considered to fuel the coping process, they are also an outcome of coping' (p. 313). In light of the known effects of daily hassles upon health, theoretical clarification of these issues is essential.

Similarly, while cognitive appraisal may implicitly involve the impact of personality variables, such as Type A behaviour and locus of control, these factors are not explicitly incorporated in the model. Recently Hobfoll (1989), in line with the perceptual nature of this model, pointed out that some people with particularly strong coping resources may not perceive stressors as such. He suggests therefore, that many stressors and the strategies used to deal with them may be lost in an overly appraised model. The focus he advocates seems to be on individuals' maintenance or conservation of their resources; however, it is difficult to see how this clearly diverges from minimizing the gap between demands and resources.

Also implied but not directly testable by the cognitive model is the dynamic nature of primary and secondary appraisals such that the resources and responses that a person can call upon in times of stress also change over time, as will the actual appraisal of harm. It is worthwhile to revisit a cybernetic model of stress proposed some years ago by Cummings and Cooper (1979) for a broader more dynamic conceptualization of these factors.

Cybernetic (or systems) model of stress

'Cybernetics is concerned with the use of information and feedback to control purposeful behavior' (Cummings and Cooper, 1979, p. 396) and maintain the organism's equilibrium. Although such a concept of homeostasis is not new (see Cannon, Selye above), it is important to appreciate that as well as the information and feedback needed by the system to achieve this, it must, by definition, also incorporate a temporal or dynamic aspect.

Miller (1965) distinguished between appraisals of stress (those factors currently affecting the individual) and of threat (those likely to have an effect in the future). The dynamic nature of a cybernetic model, through its information and feedback loops, enables both current and future demands on and resources of the system to be assessed and moderated. For instance, future demands can be prioritized, delegated, or even refused, based upon assessment of current and evolving demands and resources. However, personality, workplace, and other environmental variables will all contribute to the feedback loop.

Cummings and Cooper (1979) reviewed the literature on differences amongst individuals in their ability to cope or, in cybernetic terminology, achieve homeostasis. Type A behaviour seems 'evoked by environmental cues which threaten the individual's sense of control' (p. 402) while anxious people seem to require more feedback in order to understand and bring structure to a situation. Whilst these examples are not all-embracing, they clearly represent the import of 'personality variables' to both the appraisal and the subsequent feedback loop. Attempts to resource the situation, together with positive and negative coping strategies and environmental influences such as those input through the workplace, will also feed into the system and fluctuate over time.

It seems there is a continuous monitoring process occurring, whether at an entirely conscious and/or partly unconscious level. In Cummings and Cooper's terms, this ongoing process will inform the individual's adjustment process. In line with the general tendency to express stress outcome (or adjustment) negatively, they separate this outcome into three discrete categories: (1) indicators of strain (e.g. rapid pulse, job dissatisfaction), (2) adjustment processes (e.g. smoking, escapist drinking), and (3) long-term effects of ineffective coping (e.g. raised blood pressure).

A criticism of this model which the authors themselves posit, is the possibility of a time lag between action and feedback and further action. As this is often the nature of the world and almost certainly of the world of work, it is difficult to see how this factor can be controlled.

Implicit, but not directly assessed, amongst the variables within an individual's cybernetic feedback loop is the impact of the home environment. Moore and Cooper (1996) suggested that the interface between the person and both the work and home environments is essential to further understanding of stress and coping – or, in the terms of this model, stress and adjustment.

The Minnesota theory of work adjustment (Dawis and Lofquist, 1984), originally a primarily descriptive approach to the person–environment fit model, has itself dynamically evolved to incorporate the process of adjustment that necessarily occurs in a system. Like Cummings and Cooper, Dawis and Lofquist now state that individuals and their environments are continually adjusting to 'fit' with each other. In 1984, they outlined the various adjustment styles they considered important:

(1) Flexibility – the level of tolerance both individuals and environments have for mismatches between abilities and ability requirements, or between needs, interests, and values.
(2) Activeness – for the individual this involves changing the environment to achieve a better fit, while for the environment it involves changing the individual.
(3) Reactiveness – where either the individual or the environment acts on itself to bring about necessary changes.
(4) Perseverance – how long the individuals continue to try and improve adjustment using either active or reactive styles.

As it examines individuals' needs, values, and interests, as well as skills and reinforcers from self and job, the Minnesota theory of work adjustment may also be useful in assessing individuals' adjustment during times of transition from one lifestyle to another. It is certainly important for its conceptual engagement of both employees and employers in the 'adjustment' process.

MEASUREMENT OF INTERACTIVE COMPONENTS OF STRESS, STRAIN, ENVIRONMENT, AND PERSONALITY

This section will focus upon the Occupational Stress Indicator (OSI) (Cooper, Sloan and Williams, 1988), a comprehensive measure of *stress*, including workplace stressors (e.g. organizational structure, 61 items), strategies used to cope with stress (e.g. social support, 28 items), general behaviour (including Type A behaviour, 14 items, and locus of control, 12 items), and on the *strain* side of the equation it assesses the individual's current state of health, both mental and physical (16 items), and job satisfaction (including relationships with others, 22 items).

Although home environment is not a specific factor within the OSI, several questions are directed towards assessing its effect upon the person at work and, conversely, the effect of work demands upon the person at home. The sources of stress and the individual personality traits and coping strategies were synthesized from reviews of previous literature and are summarized in Figure 1.1 (reproduced from Robertson, Cooper and Williams, 1990). The OSI was originally designed to assess stress/strain in white-collar workers; however, recent investigations have embraced blue-collar workers.

Internal reliability and construct validity of the OSI for white-collar workers

The internal reliability (Cronbach α) and construct validity of four of the OSI's subscales – job satisfaction, health, locus of control, and Type A behaviour – were tested using multi-method multi-trait matrices with a sample of 105 management

SITUATION PERSON OUTCOMES

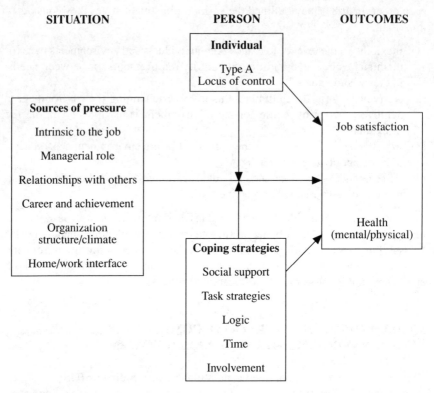

Figure 1.1 Conceptual basis for OSI.

consultants (Robertson *et al.*, 1990). While all of the sample completed the OSI during an in-house training session, only 58 employees subsequently returned the second questionnaire package designed to assess validity.

Internal reliability for job satisfaction (0.85), mental health (0.88), and physical health (0.78) were each acceptable according to Anastasi's criteria (≥ 0.7) (Anastasi, 1969); however, internal consistency for Type A was borderline (0.68) and locus of control was weak (0.38) (all $n = 105$).

Convergent validity, where two different measures of the same construct are highly correlated, was provided via the use of: Bortner's Type A Scale (Bortner and Rosenman, 1969); Warr, Cook and Wall's (1979) job satisfaction scale (only the 16 items relating to job satisfaction were used); the Crown Crisp Experiential Index (Crown and Crisp, 1979; 24 items assessing free-floating anxiety, somatic concomitants of anxiety, and depression); and Rotter's (1966) locus of control scale. The validity coefficients were: job satisfaction $r = 0.70$; mental health $r = 0.63$; Type A behaviour $r = 0.54$; and locus of control $r = 0.30$ (all $p < 0.001$, $n = 58$). In addition to these statistically significant correlations amongst monotraits, all convergent correlations were greater than those present in the heterotrait–

heteromethod matrices with the exception of the locus of control construct, which also had low (0.38) internal reliability.

There is also some concern over the discreteness of the physical health index on the OSI, although this is not directly tested in this analysis. The physical health scale on the OSI correlated 0.57 with the Crown Crisp Experiential Index and 0.59 with the OSI mental health scale. Examination of items from each of the OSI health scales does suggest some commonalities that may reflect anxiety or neuroticism. As Roberston and colleagues themselves suggest, the locus of control and physical health scale require further investigation. Despite this caveat, the components of the OSI tested by Robertson and colleagues appear to be both reliable and valid.

Internal reliability and construct validity of the OSI for blue-collar workers

Cooper and Williams (1991) adopted a similar methodology to test internal consistency and convergent reliabilities with a sample of blue-collar workers from a large chemical plant in the north-west of England ($n = 31$). Internal reliabilities of the four subscales tested were moderate to good: job satisfaction (0.88); mental health (0.87); Type A behaviour (0.67); locus of control (0.64); and physical health (0.79). Convergent validity using the same scales as Robertson and colleagues (see above) yielded values of: 0.77 for job satisfaction; 0.65 for mental health; 0.30 for Type A behaviour; and 0.36 for locus of control. All but Type A behaviour were statistically significant ≤ 0.05) and while these authors suggested that Type A behaviour may be a less salient indicator for shop-floor workers such an explanation does not explain the low heteromethod correlation.

As with white-collar workers, the OSI's physical health indicator correlated 0.40 and 0.41, respectively, with the Crown Crisp mental and somatic health scales, again suggesting that the OSI may be tapping into some more general anxiety dimension. A separate measure of neuroticism used as a covariant in future analysis would help to distinguish between these two health scales.

Empirical use of the OSI

Cooper and colleagues have utilized the OSI in several organizational stress audits and research, amassing normative data from some 14,500 persons across a range of occupations and cultures. Some major findings emanating from its use are presented below.

Health workers' profiles ($n = 1147$) compared with the bank of OSI normative data ($n = 6326$) revealed they reported significantly greater pressure from work factors such as 'managerial role', 'relationships with other people', 'career and achievement', 'organizational design and structure', and the 'home–work interface', although 'factors intrinsic to the job' were not different (Rees and Cooper, 1992). Health care workers reported greater use of all coping strategies such as social support, logic, time management, and had fewer symptoms of mental ill-health. They also reported less perceived control, congruent with high job stress, and less type A behaviour. This last finding adds to the increasingly equivocal nature of the literature regarding the impact of Type A behaviour.

Rees and Cooper (1992) examined the correlations amongst self-reported sickness absence and the OSI's subscales for job satisfaction (-0.12), mental health (0.16); and physical health (0.20) (all $p < 0.001$) in a sample of 1042 district health authority workers. Validity checks on 76 employees reported versus actual days absence revealed a small (6 per cent) overestimate on self-report. These authors suggest that, whilst not all absence will be attributable to stress, these results do indicate the criterion validity of these OSI scales. However, caution should be applied in interpreting these results, as the coefficient of determination ($r^2 \leq 4$ per cent of shared variance), whilst statistically significant, does not reveal great strength of association. Clearly other variables, such as coping and social support, may play a mediating role and these variables should be considered together in a form such as structural equation modelling.

The OSI is quickly becoming the gold standard in occupational stress research (e.g. Sutherland and Cooper, 1992) because of its comprehensive approach, and an OSI.2 has been produced which is shorter and more reliable (Williams and Cooper, 1996).

FUTURE DIRECTIONS

Current studies are moving towards the use of structural equation modelling to explain causal effects, indirect paths, and mediating effects of variables on stress. Whilst such an approach will increase our understanding of factors already under consideration, future directions in stress models might be better served by following Bacharach and Bamberger's (1992) recommendation to focus on more situation-specific or occupation-specific factors, an approach, perhaps unwittingly, often utilized in the assessment of major components of stress models. For instance, situation-specific locus of control questionnaires, self-efficacy, and coping checklists already exist. Such a situation-specific-person-specific model may yield greater understanding of the organizational climate and the changes needed in that area as well as providing insight into useful therapies for individuals. Some move towards this is already evident in the accumulation of data and the comparison of 'population profiles' being undertaken by Cooper and colleagues in the UK.

Another important dimension to be considered in future investigations is lack of positive reinforcement or *recognition for good work* as a source of dissatisfaction or stress (Moore and Cooper, 1996) and, in Selye's and Lazarus' terms, respectively, the impact of *eustress* and the *appraisal of challenge*. Are these simply what we experience before we become overburdened or are they qualitatively different? Kobasa (1979) describes the properties of people 'hardy to stress' as commitment, challenge and control, to which Moore and Burrows (1996) added communication and cognition to yield the '5 Cs'. However, it still remains unclear whether these '5 Cs' represent a mediating factor to stress or whether they may in fact equal eustress of the appraisal of challenge.

SUMMARY

This chapter has examined the evolution of stress theories from stimuli and strain to the current interactive and dynamic models. An overview of methods of assessment related to each model, their strengths and limitations, has been presented. The importance of examining both sides of the equation – stressor and strain – has been emphasized. It is suggested that a more situation-specific approach from an organizational perspective as well as that of the individual may enrich future understanding and better facilitate successful intervention programmes. The theoretical clarification of whether eustress and the appraisal of challenge are unidimensional or orthogonal to stress will also be important to future intervention strategies.

REFERENCES

Anastasi, A. (1969) *Psychological testing*, Macmillan, London.

Appley, M.H. and Trumbull, R. (1967) *Psychological stress*, Appleton Century Crofts, New York.

Bacharach, S. and Bamberger, P. (1992) Causal models of role stressor antecedents and consequents: the importance of occupational differences. *Journal of Vocational Behaviour*, **41** (1), 13–34.

Bortner, R.W. and Rosenman, R.H. (1969) The measurement of pattern A behavior. *Journal of Chronic Disease*, **20**, 525–33.

Cannon, W. (1932) *The wisdom of the body*, Norton, New York.

Cooper, C.L., Sloan, S.J. and Williams, S. (1988) *Occupational Stress Indicator: Management Guide*, NFER-Nelson, Windsor.

Cooper, C.L. and Williams, J. (1991) A validation study of the OSI on a blue collar sample. *Stress Medicine*, **7**, 109–12.

Cox, T. (1978) *Stress*. Macmillan, London.

Crown, S. and Crisp, A.H. (1979) *Manual of the Crown Crisp Experiential Index*. Hodder and Stoughton, London.

Cummings, T.G. and Cooper, C.L. (1979) A cybernetic framework for studying occupational stress. *Human Relations*, **32**, 395–418.

Dawis, R.V. and Lofquist, L.H. (1984) *A Psychological Theory of Work Adjustment: An Individual Differences Model and Its Applications*. University of Minnesota Press, Minnesota.

Dohrenwend, B.S., Krasnoff, L., Askenasy, A.R. and Dohrenwend, B.P. (1978) Exemplification of a method for scaling life events: the PERI Life Events Scale. *Journal of Health and Social Behaviour*, **19**, 205–29.

Frankenhaeuser, M. (1991) The psychophysiology of sex differences as related to occupational status, in *Women, work and health: Stress and opportunities* (eds M. Frankenhaeuser, U. Lundberg and M.A. Chesney), Plenum, New York, pp. 39–61.

Frankenhaeuser, M. (1993) Current issues on psychobiological stress research. Proceedings of the III European Congress of Psychology, Tampere, Finland.

Frankenhaeuser, M. and Gardell, B. (1976) Underload and overload in working life: outline of a multidisciplinary approach. *Journal of Human Stress*, **2**, 35–46.

Goldberg, E.L. and Comstock, G.W. (1980) Epidemiology of life events: frequency in general populations. *American Journal of Epidemiology*, **111**, 736–52.

Hobfoll, S.E. (1989) Conservation of resources: a new attempt at conceptualizing stress. *American Psychologist*, **44**, 513–24.

Holland, J.L. (1973) *Making vocational choices: A theory of careers*. Prentice-Hall, Englewood Cliffs, NJ.

Holmes, T.H. and Rahe, R.H. (1967) The social readjustment rating scale. *Journal of Psychosomatic Research*, **11**, 213–18.

Karasek, R.A. (1979) Job demands, job decision latitude and mental strain: implications for job redesign. *Administrative Science Quarterly*, **24**, 285–308.

Karasek, R., Baker, D., Marxer, F. *et al.* (1981) Job decision latitude, job demands and cardiovascular disease: a prospective study of Swedish males. *American Journal of Public Health*, **71**, 694–705.

Karasek, R.A. and Theorell, T., (1990) *Healthy Work: Stress, Productivity, and the Reconstruction of Working Life*, Basic Books, New York.

Kobasa, S.C. (1979) Stressful life events, personality and health: an inquiry into hardiness. *Journal of Personality and Social Psychology*, **37**, 1–11.

Krantz, D.S., Contrada, R.J. *et al.* (1988) Environmental stress and biobehavioral antecedents of coronary heart disease. *Journal of Consulting and Clinical Psychology*, **56**, 333–41.

Lazarus, R.S. (1966) *Psychological stress and the coping process*, McGraw-Hill, New York.

Lazarus, R.S. (1984) Puzzles in the study of daily hassles. *Journal of Behavioral Medicine*, **7**, 375–89.

Lazarus, R.S. and Folkman, S. (1984) *Stress, Appraisal and Coping*, Springer, New York.

Miller, J.G. (1965) Living systems: basic concepts. *Behavioral Science*, **10**, 193–237.

Moore, K.A. and Burrows, G.D. (1996) Stress and mental health, in *Handbook of stress, medicine and health* (ed. C.L. Cooper), CRC, London, pp. 87–100.

Moore, K. A. and Cooper C.L. (1996) Stress in mental health workers: a theoretical overview. *The International Journal of Social Psychiatry*, **42**, 82–89.

Parkes, K.R., Mendham, C.A. and von Rabenau, C. (1994). Social support and the demand–discretion model of job stress: tests of additive and interactive effects in two samples. *Journal of Vocational Behavior*, **44**, 91–113.

Rees, D.W. and Cooper, C.L. (1992) Occupational stress in health service workers in the UK. *Stress Medicine*, **8**, 79–80.

Robertson, I.R., Cooper, C.L. and Williams, J. (1990) The validity of the occupational stress indicator. *Work and Stress*, **4**, 29–39.

Ross, R.R. and Altmaier, E.M. (1994) *Intervention in occupational stress: A handbook of counselling for stress at work*, Sage Publications, London.

Rotter, J.B. (1966) Generalised expectancies for internal versus external control of reinforcement. *Psychological Monographs*, **80** (609), 1–28.

Sarason, I.G., Johnson, J.H. and Siegel, J.M. (1978) Assessing the impact of life changes: development of the Life Experiences Survey. *Journal of Consulting and Clinical Psychology*, **46**, 932–46.

Selye, H.J. (1956) *The Stress of Life*. McGraw Hill, New York.

Sharpley, C.F. (1994) Maintenence and generalizability of laboratory-based heart rate reactivity control training. *Journal of Behavioral Medicine*, **17**, 309–29.

Shedletsky, R. and Endler, N.S. (1974) Anxiety: the state–trait model and the interaction model. *Journal of Personality*, **42**, 511–27.

Sutherland, V.J. and Cooper, C.L. (1992) Job stress, satisfaction, and mental health among general practitioners before and after introduction of new contract. *British Medical Journal*, **304**, 1545–8

Taylor, A.J.W. and Frazer, A.G. (1980) Interim report of the stress effects on the recovery teams after the Mt Erebus disaster. *New Zealand Medical Journal*, **91**, 311–12.

Warr, P., Cook, J. and Wall, T. (1979) Scales for the measurement of some work attitudes and aspects of psychological well-being. *Journal of Occupational Psychology*, **52**, 129–48.

Williams, S. and Cooper, C.L. (1996) The Occupational Stress Indicator, in *Evaluating Stress: A Book of Resources* (eds C.P. Zalaquett and R.J. Wood), SHSU Press, Texas.

2 | Stress in health professions: a review of the research literature

Sally Hardy and Ben Thomas

There are numerous articles that refer to stress and its contributory components. To cover all aspects would take more than one book, let alone one chapter. This chapter looks at stress research amongst health professionals, the most commonly used definition of stress within the research literature and some of the factors contributing to the psychological consequences of professional caring.

Although stress at work has been linked with physical and mental ill health, it largely remains seen as an individual problem or failing. People react differently to stress, and its effects can also be manifest differently. One person may suffer migraines and headaches, whilst another will suffer sleep disturbance and loss of appetite (refer to Table 2.1). These individual responses do not mean, however, that stress is an individual problem. What is becoming more clear is the interplay between the individual and the organizational level of need. Stress research has evolved and continues to evolve with the changing demands of the workplace setting. The health care arena is one of many areas that has undergone major levels of change during the last decade. Evidence is increasing towards the conclusion that stress in the workplace has national implications on health policy initiatives and developments.

STRESS AND ITS CONSEQUENCES

Whilst stress can be a product of working and caring for people, it is still an occupational hazard that can be controlled and managed like any other. Through the identification of risk factors and the introduction of appropriate measures to eliminate or control them, stress and ill health in the workplace can be drastically reduced.

Caring is a stressful occupation. Stress has consequences for the carer and implications for recipients (Bowden, 1994). There are effects on economical outcomes such as loss of productivity through absenteeism, industrial relations problems, poor decision making, low morale, and an increased risk of work accidents (Sutherland and Cooper, 1992). Stress is attributed to health problems from minor ailments, such as headaches and migraines, through to life threatening diseases, such as heart disease and cancers (Cox, 1978). A MIND report (MIND, 1992) found that 21 per cent of all companies approached believed sickness rates were a direct result of stress-related health problems.

STRESS, WHEN EMOTIONS HURT

Derived from the Latin word, *stringere* (to draw tight), 'stress' has become a word that is widely used but often with little thought of the complex models and implications with which stress has become associated. Hinkle (1973) covers the fascinating evolution of concepts of stress through history and that publication is used as an introduction to research developments in Cooper (1996). As can be seen from Table 2.1, stress has consequences for the carer.

Most theoretical models suggest that stress results from demands outstripping resources, which sounds simple enough but does not include the intrinsic and external influences that interfere and complicate (Bowden, 1994). In the work setting, stress has been described as a result of job demands being influenced by individual and environmental characteristics (Cooper and Payne, 1988). For example Cherniss (1980), Maslach (1982), and Hood (1985) suggest that stress results from the demands of caring mediated by aspects of work setting and the resources available to individuals to carry out their job successfully. The Health Education Authority (1988) defines stress as an excess demand on an individual beyond their capability to cope. All are similar definitions of the same stress model but represent very different components of the same thing, i.e. occupational stress.

Little research has been carried out, however, on the collective or contagious effect of stress. The study of stress at work would benefit from attention to the ways in which people shape their environment to protect themselves in order to facilitate or stunt growth and activity (Bunce and West, 1994).

Methodological problems with stress studies according to Cushway (1992) are largely threefold: (a) inadequate comparison and clear use of operational definitions for stress; (b) lack of clarity in defining what are stress related problems and then; (c) a reliance on subjective descriptions of stress. Despite these criticisms, Nathan (1986) believes that self report measures of stress can provide reliable and valid data, whilst personal descriptions of the more complex interactional conceptualizations of stress is becoming a more widely recognized method of data collection within naturalistic research methods (Barlow, Hayes and Nelson, 1984; Schon, 1983).

Table 2.1 Stress in the public sector (adapted from: Health Education Authority, 1988).

Behavioural	Physical	Emotional
Short term		
Overindulgence and reliance on smoking, drinking alcohol, or drug taking	Headaches	Tiredness/irritability
Increased risk of accidents	Backache	Anxiety
Impulsive/reactionary behaviour	Poor/disturbed sleep pattern	Boredom
Poor relationships with others at home and at work	Indigestion	Depression/mood swings
Apathy	Chest pain Nausea Dizziness	Inability to concentrate Low self-esteem
Long term		
Marital breakdown	Heart disease	Insomnia
Social isolation	Hypertension Ulcers Poor general health	Chronic depression and anxiety Neurosis Suicide

BURNOUT

Maslach and Jackson (1981) conceptualized burnout as a pattern of emotional over-load and exhaustion resulting from working in the caring professions. Burnout is considered to reveal itself in feelings of emotional exhaustion, a sense of being drained of energy and motivation. Maslach (1982) proposed that if burnout is allowed to continue unheeded, individuals are at risk of becoming detached from their work as a way of coping. In addition individuals will feel they are not achiev-ing or accomplishing anything, which in itself will lead to feelings of low self-worth.

Maslach and Jackson (1981) developed the Maslach Burnout Inventory (MBI) to measure the three components: emotional exhaustion, depersonalization, and reduced feelings of personal achievement. Burnout has also been extensively covered by Cherniss (1980), who viewed the process as principally arising from the intrinsic demands of caring for people in distress, which can eventually lead to job strain.

As a result, burnout has been studied extensively throughout the helping pro-fessions (Freudenberger, 1975; Pines and Maslach, 1978; Payne and Firth-Cozens, 1987; Caton et al., 1988; Edwards and Miltenberger, 1991). However, much of the work is descriptive, lacks a clear theoretical basis, and typically looks at single aspects of burnout.

Although Maslach's three-factor model is the most widely used, there are other operational definitions cited in the literature. In a review of work organizations,

Shirom (1989) concludes that the various models of burnout share three common features. First burnout describes an individual phenomenon, second it is a negative experience, and third it is chronic and ongoing. However, there is much left open to debate. The concept has been defined as a unidimensional model based upon the core components of physical and mental exhaustion (Garden, 1987), although evidence remains based largely upon descriptive studies and is therefore inconclusive (Evans and Fischer, 1993). Perhaps more interestingly, researchers have avoided cross-referencing work on burnout with stress, largely because stress is not considered necessarily a negative or chronic experience (Bradley and Sutherland, 1995). Stress models that are stimulus based and consider stress and burnout a result of external influences on the individual deny the influence of more intrinsic factors. Thus stress is a complex phenomenon and any model should take into consideration not only the individual but also the environmental, dynamic, and interactive nature of stress (Sutherland and Cooper, 1992).

There is some evidence that burnout can be linked with depression (Firth *et al.*, 1987); hence depression has become another measure obtained through the use of Beck's Depression Inventory (Beck and Beck, 1972) when considering levels of burnout in staff and carers. Again this link is tentative, and probably exists at the latter end of the burnout continuum, if stress is left unnoticed and unattended.

COPING STRATEGIES

A common assumption of early research studies (e.g. Selye, 1936) is that individuals cope by adapting themselves to stressful environments. This led to interest in coping styles as a means of measuring individuals' response to stress.

Lazarus and Folkman (1984) define coping as a person's constantly changing cognitive and behavioural efforts to manage the specific environmental and/or internal demands that are placed upon them. This structure distinguishes at a general level between problem-focused and emotion-regulating coping. Difference in coping style has been used to account for individuals' different means of adapting to stress at various levels. Cherniss (1980) saw active problem solving as a positive coping mechanism to help deal with caring, although its overall effect on patients and society as a whole remains to be seen.

In their model Lazarus and Folkman (1984) propose that coping strategies are chosen in response to an event and influence adaptation. They distinguish between problem-focused and emotionally focused coping strategies. Problem-focused strategies are directed towards the management of problems whilst emotionally focused responses involve a failure to confront the problem, dealing instead with emotional distress. There is some evidence to suggest that concentrating on the emotionally focused response has a negative effect on well-being (Israel *et al.*, 1989).

The experience of stress need not be negative, so coping styles or strategies are considered as mediating influences (Bradley and Sutherland, 1995). Coping techniques may influence the interaction between the individual and their environment, thus changing the individual's understanding and their response to a stressful situation (Dewe and Guest, 1990).

Lazarus and Folkman's (1984) cognitive–phenomenological model of stress and coping has guided many further studies on the direct effect of personal and social resources, appraisals, and coping upon levels of psychological adjustment (Cronin-Stubbs and Brophy, 1985; Ceslowitz, 1989). The central theme is how events are appraised by the individual as stressful and whether the stress exceeds a person's coping resources and skills (Callan and Terry, 1994). Researchers have typically distinguished between personal and social resources, with those people having higher self-esteem more likely to have a history of coping effectively under stress (Holahan and Moos, 1987; Ashford, 1988). Individuals considered to function with an internal locus of control adapt better to stressful situations than those with an external locus of control (Callan and Dickson, 1992).

Ceslowitz (1989) random sample of hospital nurses revealed that those nurses who used the coping strategies of escape/avoidance, self-controlling and confronting experienced greater levels of burnout than those nurses who coped using strategies of problem-solving, positive reappraisal and seeking social support. Which led her to conclude that it was the cognitive appraisal of a situation that led to the person's ability to deal with stress.

Attributional styles have received most attention in literature in connection with learnt helplessness and depression (Bowden, 1994). Abramson, Seligman and Teasdale (1978) proposed that internal and global explanations for events contribute to depression. Brewin (1985) supports this suggestion in that one's sense of control over negative events in relation to oneself can contribute to depression. This has led to studies on the assumption that personal control over working conditions is linked with positive or negative health outcomes (Spillane, 1980; Warr, 1987). Therefore the topic of negative events at work in relation to attributional style is an area of interest in occupational stress research.

SUPPORT; A FRIEND INDEED

Cherniss (1980) found that those individuals with significant and rewarding relationships outside work seemed to suffer less from work strain. Life events outside work are considered likely to affect a person's ability to cope at work; several studies conclude that individuals suffering depression are more likely to be going through external life events (Thompson and Hendrie, 1972; Brown and Harris, 1978; Power and Champion, 1992).

Cohen and Willis (1985) argued that the effects of social support vary as a function of the type of measure of support being used. For example, the size or extent of social support can be considered to equate with an individual's sense of belonging, the perceived supportiveness of the network acting as a buffer to the negative effects of stress. Studies on the role of social support have tended to find little or no evidence of a buffering effect but actually report that availability of social support exacerbated negative effects (Israel *et al.*, 1989).

Social support is embedded in ongoing social interactions (Buunk and Hoorens, 1992). Buunk (1990) identified four conceptions of social support from the occupational stress literature. First, a sociological perspective: social support is seen as the number of connections an individual has with others, or the size of one's social network. Second, social support can be equated with the availability of satisfying relationships characterised by love, intimacy, trust, or esteem. Cutrona and Russell (1990) reveal that successful relationships, ones that provide attachment, belonging and a reassurance of one's self-worth, can act as a buffer to stress. Third, the perceived helpfulness of social support constitutes the appraisal that under stressful circumstances others can be relied upon for support, advice, empathetic understanding, and guidance (Sarason and Sarason, 1986). And finally, the concept of social support refers primarily to the actual receiving of supportive acts from others once a stressful situation comes into existence. Despite this differentiation, the role of social support on the negative or positive outcome of stress remains inconclusive. Buunk and Hoorens (1992) go on to discuss in detail all aspects of social support and conclude with no clearer definitions of the effect of social support on stress. The beneficial effects of social support are that situations that arise should not be taken for granted and that tailor-made responses cannot be defined as each situation will warrant different responses.

Moos (1976) theorized that people are more satisfied and tend to perform better in an environment where interpersonal relationships are emphasized. One way in which this has been actualized is through staff support or sensitivity groups. Groups within the workplace setting provide a structure where staff are encouraged to meet together to share their work experience, listen to each other and provide shared opportunity for learning and developing through problem solving and support (see for example Bion, 1961; Yalom, 1975).

Feinbloom and Brod (1986) found that staff who participated in groups experienced less emotional exhaustion as compared to a control group. Bernstein Hyman (1993) also studied staff groups working in long-term geriatric settings, who were exposed to three 3-hour group sessions and found significant benefits for all staff involved.

Blauner (1964) and Seeman (1959) found isolation from work colleagues as having a negative effect on work competence and Cherniss (1980) found physical and psychological availability of co-workers were being used as a compensation for poor supervision. These elements cannot be expanded upon here, but are taken up again within other chapters in the book.

We turn now to two of the largest professions working within the health care arena, but by no means the most important. Research into occupational stress has been carried out in these two areas, although significance can be seen to other health disciplines.

NURSES

Menzies (1959) was probably the first to identify the effects of caring on nurses. Her study of a London teaching hospital graphically described how nurses are affected by the emotional impact of caring for distressed people. The work environment arouses strong emotional responses in the nurse which range from compassion and pity to anger and resentment. By the very nature of their work, nurses are therefore at risk of being overcome with anxiety. They respond using defence mechanisms that lead to avoidance behaviour (avoiding contact with patients, decision making, and responsibilities) and the denial of feelings, which leads to depersonalization. Menzies concluded that although these social defence mechanisms were necessary to ensure the institutions continued in their primary function of providing care, little or no attention was paid to helping nurses deal with or even recognize their anxiety.

In a contemporary study, Meerbeau (1986) identified that stress could be revealed in some of the difficulties associated with a largely female workforce, as is evident with nurses. Women are more likely to be juggling the responsibilities of home life, families and careers. Insufficient child care arrangements and an increase in the elderly population as a whole mean that nurses are more likely to be involved as primary carer both in and out of the work situation. Meerbeau also revealed how nurses who work part time are overlooked for promotion. Cooper and Melhuish (1982) revealed that women at management level were concerned about coping with work pressures and complained of feeling irritable and having bouts of anxiety, tiredness, anger, and sleep disturbance. Tschudin (1985) reported on how nurses felt insecure in their long-term career path due to the immense rate of change within the health service and that individualized health care provision meant nurses could not provide the care they wished due to lack of resources. Providing emotional care to patients was not considered important nor were nurses encouraged to identify and deal with their emotions (Booth, 1988).

A number of studies have attempted to assess the extent of stress on the mental health of nurses and other outcome measures. Tyler *et al.* (1991) reported significant correlations between a Nursing Stress Scale (Gray-Toft and Anderson, 1981) and the GHQ (Goldberg, 1978). In another study Tyler and Cushway (1992) reported two main factors identified by hospital-based nurses. One factor was the physical environment and the structure of their work – in other words, lack of staff, conflicting time pressures and demands, and perceived lack of resources and equipment. The second factor was the problem of dealing with dying patients and their relatives, which was often linked with a feeling there was inadequate preparation and support for nurses in dealing with death. Tyler and Cushway (1992) conclude their study by recommending organizational support for nurses through the provision of stress management packages targeting the learning of new coping strategies, and in-service training and workshops.

Nurses have been identified as having high suicide and psychiatric referral rates (Jones *et al.*, 1987) and high incidence of smoking, alcohol and drug-taking habits

(Plant, Plant and Foster, 1992). The number of nurses reported as leaving the profession due to stress is grossly underestimated. Many nurses leave the profession prior to qualifying (Murray, Swan and Mathau, 1983), whilst others leave as a result of stress in their work setting. Few studies have addressed the relationship between stress, burnout and turnover or absenteeism (Bowden, 1994). Jackson *et al.* (1986) found emotional exhaustion correlated with job turnover, within a twelve month study period. Lazaro *et al.* (1985) reported links between alienation and burnout to job turnover or an intention to leave. Surveys of the opinions of psychiatric nurses, who reveal that 'leavers' were statistically shown to be more dissatisfied with their job, the quality of decision making, in-service training, physical work conditions, and scored higher on the burnout scale (Cherniss, 1980) and were younger, less experienced, but more highly qualified than 'stayers'. The continuing concerns about a shortage of qualified nurses have led to speculation that nursing as a profession might cease to exist by the year 2000.

MEDICS

Firth-Cozens (1987) identified gender difference in stress levels amongst medical staff. Female general practitioners (GPs) exhibited more free-floating anxiety and depression than their male colleagues (Sutherland and Cooper, 1992) whilst almost half the female junior doctors studied were considered clinically depressed. A principal contributory factor for female doctors is the conflict between family and career (Bynoe, 1994). One suggestion is that because late evenings and extensive overtime are impossible for women with families, this acts as a buffer to additional stress. Alongside this there is increasing evidence that married female doctors are less stressed than single ones, which is contrary to the situation for the general public (Bynoe, 1993). In general, women have been found to report psychological distress at a higher rate than have men (Davidson and Cooper, 1986).

Caplan (1994) studied stress, anxiety, and depression in a group of senior health service staff (81 hospital consultants, 322 GPs and 121 senior hospital managers). Using the General Health Questionnaire (GHQ, Goldberg and Williams, 1988) and a hospital depression and anxiety questionnaire, he showed that senior medical staff (i.e. consultants and GPs) were considerably more likely to be suffering from depression than senior managers, whilst GPs were significantly more likely to have suicidal thoughts. He concludes that, although senior medical staff suffered from high levels of stress, senior managers revealed similarly high stress levels but manifest in different ways. Stress research had previously concentrated on junior medical staff but this study identified stress occurring at all levels within the health care arena.

Bradley and Sutherland (1995) surveyed social workers and home helps to find statistical correlation of the suggestion that work stress was having an adverse effect on the health of social service workers. Both groups identified emotional and physical exhaustion as among the most frequent symptoms experienced. Although exhaustion is normally considered an element of burnout, burnout was not an item specifically measured in this study. The results were gathered from an isolated sample population. A questionnaire was developed for the purpose of the research carried out to identify the needs of a stress management programme. The results are considered by the authors to be applicable more widely.

Parallels have been drawn between professional and informal carers in their suffering of stress and burnout as a result of caring for others. Hoenig and Hamilton (1967) made a distinction between the subjective and objective burden experienced by carers of elderly people. Objective burden was considered to be the adverse effects on the household such as loss of earnings and income, whilst subjective burden was the burden taken upon the relatives themselves. Burden has some connection with burnout (Bowden, 1994), although little research has been carried out in this area.

CONCLUSION

There is growing realization that the subject of stress is best approached as a mental construct and a result of several interacting phenomena (Gregson and Looker, 1994). Gregson and Looker (1994) propose a mind and body interactive model of stress (Figure 2.1) which they believe aids the implementation of effective stress management programmes (Figure 2.2).

Concern today centres around the effect of immense change in the workplace, leading to inevitable reorganization, relocation, redefinition of roles and responsibilities, and an increased amount of stress. Fewer people are employed to carry out the work, exerting enormous pressure upon the slimline work force that remains (Cooper, 1996).

According to Cooper (1996) the first and most effective way of dealing with stress is to eliminate its source. This may involve considerable and controversial measures, such as redefining job descriptions, devolving decision making, and policy development. Training and education programmes are important in helping people develop their style of work and their mechanisms for coping with stress. One of these might be an organization-wide acceptance of confidential counselling. Overall, therefore, stress is best managed at both individual and organizational levels.

The overall impression from the literature is that stress is complex and dynamic in nature. Research into stress and its components continues to flourish and yet has remained restricted by the methodological and design problems of population studies and of obtaining accurate tools of measurement. There does not appear to be much progress in further understanding the complexities of occupational stress (Bradley and Sutherland, 1995). Yet one of the most intriguing aspects of stress is that it is revealing its complexity alongside new knowledge. Consideration of the serious repercussions of occupational stress for those involved in health care delivery is beginning to evolve at policy-making levels.

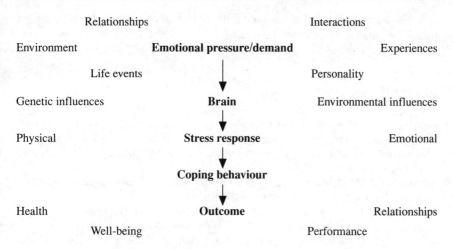

Figure 2.1 A whole body and mind interactive model of stress. Adapted from Gregson and Looker (1994).

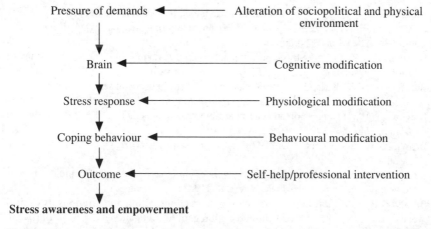

Figure 2.2 A model for stress management and intervention. Adapted from Gregson and Looker (1994).

Stress amongst staff is becoming a major concern to employers as the cost of caring rises not only in monetary terms but also in terms of the efficiency of the services provided. The Health Education Authority and the NHS management executive have both recommended promoting health at work. The British Medical Association has launched a 24 hour emergency telephone helpline for doctors suffering stress that might jeopardize their professional work. The accumulation of research, however small the sample group, has led to a considerable body of evidence to suggest not only to individual health care workers how debilitating stress at work can be, but also that national initiatives are beginning to recognize their role in helping the carers continue to care.

REFERENCES

Abramson, L., Seligman, M. and Teasdale, J. (1978) Learned helplessness in humans: critique and reformulation. *Journal of Abnormal Psychology*, **87**, 49–74.

Alexander, D.A. (1993) Staff support groups: do they support and are they even groups? *Palliative Medicine*, **7**, 127–32.

Ashford, S.J. (1988) Individual strategies for coping with stress during organisational transition. *The Journal of Applied Behavioural Science*, **24**, 19–36.

Barlow, D.H., Hayes, S.C. and Nelson, R.O. (1984) *The Scientist Practitioner. Research and accountability in clinical and educational settings*. Allyn and Bacon, MA, USA.

Beck, A.T. and Beck, R.W. (1972) Screening depressed patients in family practice: a rapid technique. *Postgraduate Medical*, **52**, 81–5.

Bernstein Hyman, R. (1993) Evaluation of an intervention for staff in long term care facility using a retrospective pretest design. *Evaluation and the Health Professions*, **16** (2), 212–24.

Bion, W.R. (1961) *Experiences in Groups*. Tavistock Publications, London.

Blauner, R. (1964) *Alienation and Freedom*, University of Chicago Press, Chicago.

Booth, K. (1988) Stress and nurses. *Nursing*, **3** (30), 1017–20.

Bowden, G. (1994) Work stress, burnout and coping. A review and an empirical study of staff supported housing. *Clincial Psychology and Psychotherapy*, **1** (4), 219–32.

Bradley, J. and Sutherland, V. (1995) Occupational stress in social services: a comparison of social workers and home help staff. *British Journal of Social Work*, **25**, 313–31.

Brewin, C. (1985) Depression and causal attributions: what is their relation? *Psychological Bulletin*, **98**, 297–309.

Brown, G.W. and Harris, T.O. (1978) *Social Origins of Depression*, Tavistock Press, London.

Bunce, D. and West, M. (1994) Changing work environments: innovative coping responses to occupational stress. *Work and Stress*, **8**, 319–31.

Buunk, B.P. (1990) Affiliation and helping interactions within organisations. A critical analysis of the role of social support with regard to occupational stress, in *European Review of Social Psychology* (eds W. Stroebe and M. Hewstone), Vol. 1, John Wiley, Chichester, pp. 293–322.

Buunk, B.P. and Hoorens, V. (1992) Social support and stress: the role of social comparison and social exchange processes. *British Journal of Clinical Psychology*, **31**, 445–57.

Bynoe, A.G. (1993) *Will she won't she?* A study into career decision making and its consequences in women doctors. Dissertation for Diploma in Health Services Management. University of York.

Bynoe, A.G. (1994) Stress in women doctors. *British Journal of Hospital Medicine*, **51**, 267–9.

Callan, V.J. and Dickson, C. (1992) Managerial coping strategies during organisational change. *Asia-Pacific Journal of Human Resources*, **30**, 47–59.

Callan, V. J. and Terry, D.J. (1994) Coping resources, coping strategies and adjustment to organisational change: direct or buffering effects. *Work and Stress*, **8**, 372–83.

Caplan, R.P. (1994) Stress, anxiety and depression in hospital consultants, general practitioners and senior health service managers. *British Medical Journal*, **309**, 1261–3.

Ceslowitz, S.B. (1989) Burnout and coping strategies among hospital staff nurses. *Journal of Advanced Nursing*, **14**, 553–7.

Cherniss, C. (1980) *Staff burnout. Job stress in Humans Services*, Sage Publications, Beverly Hills.

Cohen, S. and Willis, T.A. (1985) Stress, social support and the buffering hypothesis. *Psychological Bulletin*, **98**, 310–57.

Cooper, C. (1996) Stress in the workplace. *British Journal of Hospital Medicine*, **55** (9), 559–63.

Cooper, C. and Melhuish, A. (1982) Can women take pressure? *The Times*, 17 February.

Cooper, C.L. and Payne, R. (1988) *Causes, coping and consequences of stress at work*, John Wiley, Chichester.

Cox, T. (1978) *Stress*, Macmillan Education, London.

Cronin-Stubbs, D. and Brophy, E.B. (1985) Burnout. Can social support save the psych nurse? *Journal of Psychosocial Nursing*, **23** (7), 8–13.

Cushway, D. (1992) Stress in clinical psychology trainees. *British Journal of Clinical Psychology*, **31**, 169–79.

Cutrona, C. and Russell, D. (1990) Type of social support and specific stress: Toward a theory of optimal matching, in *Social Support: An Interactional View* (eds B.R. Sarason, I.G. Sarason and G.R. Pierce), New York. Wiley.

Davidson, M.J. and Cooper, C.L. (1986) *Shattering the Glass Ceiling. The Woman Manager*, Paul Chapman Publishing, London.

Dewe, P.J. and Guest, D. (1990) Methods of coping with stress at work; a conceptual analysis and empirical study of measurement issues. *Journal of Organisational Behaviour*, **11**, 135–50.

Doyle, D. (1986) Staff stress: prevention and management, in *Terminal Care* (ed. R. Turnbull), Hemisphere Publishing Group, Washington.

Edwards, P. and Miltenberger, R. (1991) Burnout among staff members at community residential facilities for persons with mental retardation. *Mental Retardation*, **29**, 125–8.

Evans, B.K. and Fischer, D.G. (1993) The nature of burnout: a study of the three factor model of burnout in human service and non human service samples. *Journal of Occupational and Organisational Psychology*, **66**, 29–38.

Feinbloom, R.I. and Brod, M.S. (1986) The functional effectiveness of nursing home patients. Unpublished manuscript. State University of New York, Stony Brook, NY.

Firth, H. *et al.* (1987) Burnout and professional depression: related concepts? *Journal of Advanced Nursing*, **11**, 633–41.

Firth-Cozens, J. (1987) Emotional distress in junior house officers. *British Medical Journal*, **295**, 533–6.

Freudenberger, H. (1975) The staff burnout syndrome in alternative institutions. *Psychotherapy: Theory, Research and Practice*, **12**, 72–83.

Garden, A.M. (1987) Depersonalisation: a valid dimension of burnout? *Human Relations*, **40**, 545–60.

Goldberg, D.P. (1978) *Manual of the General Health Questionniare*, NFER–Nelson, Windsor.

Goldberg, D.P. and Williams, P. (1988) *A User's Guide to the General Health Questionnaire*, NFER–Nelson, Windsor.

Gray-Toft, P. and Anderson, J.G. (1981) The nursing stress scale. Development of an instrument. *Journal of Behavioural Assessment*, **3**, 139–45.

Gregson, O. and Looker, T. (1994) The biological basis of stress management. *British Journal of Guidance and Counselling*, **22**, 13–26.

Health Education Authority (1988) Stress in the public sector. HMSO, London.

Hinkle, L.E. (1973) The concept of stress in the biological sciences. *Stress Medicine and Man*, **1**, 31–48.

Hoenig, J. and Hamilton, M. (1967) Extramural psychiatric care and the elderly. *British Journal of Psychiatry*, **113**, 435–43.

Holahan, C.J. and Moos, R.H. (1987) Personal and contextual determinants of coping strategies. *Journal of Personality and Psychological Medicine*, **9**, 139–45.

Hood, S. (1985) Staff needs, staff organisation and effective primary task performance in the residential setting. *International Journal of Therapeutic Communities*, **6** (1), 15–36.

Israel, B.A., House, J.S., Schurman, S.J. *et al.* (1989) The relation of personal resources, participation, influences, interpersonal relationships and coping strategies to occupational stress, job strain and health; a multivariate analysis. *Work and Stress*, **3**, 163–94.

Jackson, S.E., Schwas, R.L. and Schuler, R.S. (1986) Towards and understanding of the burnout phenomenon. *Journal of Applied Psychology*, **71**, 630–40.

Jones, J.G. *et al.* (1987) Some determinants of stress in psychiatric nurses. *International Journal of Nursing Studies*, **24** (2), 129–44.

Lazaro, C., Shinn, M. and Robinson, P. (1985) Burnout, job performance and withdrawal behaviours. *Journal of Health and Human Resources Administration*, **7**, 213–34.

Lazarus, R.S. and Folkman, S. (1984) *Stress, Appraisal and Coping*, Springer, New York.

Lee, F. (1995) Why sick doctors play hide and seek. *Healthcare Management*. March, 8–12.

Maslach, C. (1982) Understanding burnout: defintional issues in analysing a complex phenomenon, in *Job stress and burnout* (ed. W.S. Paine), Sage Publications, Beverly Hills, pp. 20–40.

Maslach, C. and Jackson, S.E. (1981) The measurement of experienced burnout. *Journal of Occupational Behaviour*, **2**, 99–113.

Meerbeau, L. (1986) Jobs for the girls? *Nursing Times*, 82 (**23**), 31–3.

Menzies, I.E.P. (1959) A case study in the functioning of social systems as a defence against anxiety. *Human Relations*, **13**, 95–121.

MIND (1992) *The MIND Survey: Stress at Work*, MIND: National Association for Mental Health, London.

Moos, R.H. (1976) Evaluating and changing community settings. *American Journal of Community Psychology*, **4**, 313–25.

Murray, H., Swan, A.V. and Mathau, N. (1983) The task of nursing and the risk of smoking. *Journal of Advanced Nursing*, **8**, 131–8.

Nathan, P.E. (1986) Unanswered questions about distressed professionals, in *Professionals in Distress* (eds R. Kilburg, P.E. Nahan and R.W. Thoreson), American Psychological Association, New York.

Payne, R. and Firth-Cozens, J. (1987) *Stress in Health Professionals*, John Wiley, Chichester.

Pines and Maslach (1978) Characteristics of staff turnover in mental health settings. *Hospital and Community Psychiatry*, **29**, 233–7.

Plant, M.L., Plant, M.A. and Foster, J. (1992) Stress, alcohol, tobacco and illicit drug use amongst nurses: a Scottish study. *Journal of Advanced Nursing*, **17**, 1057–67.

Power, M.J. and Champion, L.A. (1992) The Significant Other Scale (SOS), in *A Mental Health Assessment Resource Pack* (ed. D. Milne), NFER–Nelson, Windsor.

Quick, J.C. and Quick, J.D. (1984) *Organisational Stress and Preventative Management*, McGraw Hill, New York.

Sarason, I.G. and Sarason, B.R. (eds) (1986) Experimentally provided social support. *Journal of Personality and Social Psychology*, **50**, 1222–5.

Schon, D.A. (1983) *The Reflective Practitioner. How Professionals Think in Action*. Basic Books Inc., NY, USA.

Seeman, S. (1959) On the meaning of alienation. *American Sociological Review*, **24**, 738–91.

Selye, H. (1936) *Stress in Health and Disease*, Butterworth Press, Sevenoaks.

Shirom, A. (1989) Burnout in organisations, in *International review of Industrial and Organisational Psychology* (eds C.L. Cooper and I. Robertson), John Wiley, Chichester, pp. 25–48.

Spillane, R. (1980) Overseas research developments, in *Stress at work* (ed. H.L. Bartely), Symposium Series 1, La Trobe University Department of Psychology, pp. 36–52.

Sutherland, V.J. and Cooper, C.L. (1992) Job stress, satisfaction and mental health among general practitioners before and after introduction of new contract. *British Medical Journal*, **304**, 1545–8.

Thompson, K.C. and Hendrie, H.C. (1972) Environmental stress in primary depressive illness. *Archives of General Psychiatry*, **26**, 130.

Tschudin, V. (1985) Too much pressure. *Nursing Times*, **81** (37), 30–1; **81** (38), 45–6.

Tyler, P. and Cushway, D. (1992) Stress, coping and mental well-being in hospital nurses. *Stress Medicine*, **8**, 91–8.

Tyler, P.A, Carroll, D. and Cunningham, S.E. (1991) Stress and well-being in nurses. A comparison of the public and private sectors. *International Journal of Nursing Studies*, **28**, 125–30.

Warr, P. (1987) *Work, Unemployment and Mental Health*. Clarendon Press, Oxford.

Yalom, I.D. (1970) *Theory and Practice of Group Psychotherapy*. Basic Books Inc., NY, USA.

<table>
<tr><td>3</td><td># Stress and burnout in student health care professionals</td></tr>
</table>

| 3 | **Stress and burnout in student health care professionals** |

P. Joe Tobin, Vedan Gunnoo and Jerome Carson

In this chapter the literature on stress in student health and social care professionals is reviewed. A number of key empirical studies are examined in detail. The findings from two studies conducted by the authors are presented. The first is a study of stress, coping and burnout in nursing students at pre-registration and post-registration levels. The second is a study of stress, burnout and organizational commitment in social work students. The implications of the findings from these studies are highlighted, and directions for future research in this field are outlined.

INTRODUCTION

Looking back at the stresses of their own student days may be difficult for many readers with the passage of time. They may have forgotten how stressful their training actually was. They may regard today's students as being better off than they were. For instance, when one of us trained as a clinical psychologist, only three out of eight students on the masters programme for clinical psychology were actually funded. The remaining five students had to pay their own course fees, find their own living and accommodation expenses, and received no payment for three days' work per week over a three-year period in the National Health Service. Today, most clinical psychology students are paid. However, being a student health or social care professional brings with it an 'in between' status. You are not yet a qualified nurse, physiotherapist, or social worker, but someone 'in training'. Patients may even refuse to let you sit in with your supervisor. The process of training may in itself be inherently stressful. In recent years in Britain, nurse education has moved towards a bursary system of funding. Effectively this means that students are less well off financially. Standards of nursing accommodation have declined in many parts of the country. Student nurses also spend less time on the wards, which may hinder the nurse socialization process. Cumulatively, less money, poorer accommodation and less time on the ward may create greater stress in today's student nurses. Similarly, one wonders what effects the latest government pay round, in which nurses received the lowest increment of all the professional groups, may have on student nurses' morale. Equally, given the rapid speed of change in the contemporary British health service, and the stresses this inevitably puts on staff, one wonders does this stress transmit itself from qualified staff to students in training?

We need to ask the question therefore: is the process of training as a health or social care professional an intrinsically stressful one? Certainly, it is not difficult to recognize events that are stressful to students in clinical settings. At a recent staff student course meeting, students asked whether certain topics, such as suicide and rape, could be taught in a more sensitive way so as to minimize the distress they experienced. Qualified professionals often become desensitized to the stressful nature of their jobs, frequently involving matters of life and death, and hence may forget how stressful these events may be to students, some of whom may be facing these issues for the first time. Of course it could also be argued that high stress levels in students might be the result of selecting unsuitable students for training. In the guise of selecting candidates who may be more empathic, or who have greater life experiences to offer, students with more neurotic dispositions may unintentionally be chosen. In a sense this might be described as the 'nature nurture' debate of the stresses of clinical training.

STRESS IN STUDENT HEALTH AND SOCIAL CARE PROFESSIONALS: THE LITERATURE REVIEWED

A literature review using the PsycLIT database revealed 134 articles on stress in students during the period 1988–1995. Search terms were 'stress', 'occupational stress', 'psychological stress', 'social stress', 'distress', and 'stress management'. The following student groups were surveyed : college students, graduate students, medical students, postgraduate students, and vocational students. A second Medline search for the same period revealed some 367 papers. It is not the intention of the present chapter to review these exhaustively, but rather to highlight specific themes in the literature.

Perhaps not surprisingly, the greatest number of studies of stress in students have been conducted on medical students. For instance, Mosley *et al.* (1994), looked at coping, depression, stress, and somatic distress in medical students completing a psychiatric placement. They found clinical levels of depression amongst 23 per cent of the sample, with 57 per cent reporting high levels of somatic distress. Bramness, Fixdal and Vaglum (1991) compared medical students with the normal population and found they did not differ in mental health. Male students were found to have more nervous symptoms and lower self-esteem than female students.

Nursing students probably constitute the second most researched professional group. Scullion (1994) looked at stressors affecting student nurses in accident and emergency departments. Lindop (1989) examined why nurses left training as a result of stress, and interviewed a sample of 23 such leavers. Everly *et al.* (1994) conducted a national survey of stress and coping in occupational therapy students. Interestingly they found that student occupational therapists were more stressed by the academic demands of their training than by clinical concerns. Ramanaidu (1991) found that radiography students were also most stressed by their academic curriculum, but additionally noted greater distress in overseas students.

The second major type of studies concerns the measurement of stress in student populations. Several authors have attempted to validate questionnaire measures of student stress. See for instance the Graduate Stress Inventory (Rocha-Singh, 1994); the Student Life Stress Inventory (Gadzella, 1994); the College Stress Inventory (Solberg *et al.*, 1993); the Inventory of College Students' Recent Life Experiences (Kohn and Gurevich, 1993), to name but a few of these measures. The third major theme in the literature concerns how students adjusted to a different culture, or how cultural factors might be operating in the student body. An example of the former type of study is that of Sandhu (1994), who considered the specific stressors faced by foreign students, and suggests a number of strategies to reduce acculturative stress. An example of the latter is that of Cheng, Leong and Geist (1993), who compared Asian and Causcasian American undergraduates on the Brief Symptom Inventory. They found that Asians experience a greater degree of personal problems than do Causcasians. A fourth theme in the literature concerns studies that attempt to predict which factors might be related to student stress. Um and Brown-Standrige (1993) conducted interviews with social work students, and identified a number of organizational factors that were likely to increase stress. These centred around 'hierarchy', 'role', 'accountability' and 'organizational binds'. Additional themes in the research literature concern exam stress (e.g. Tooth, Tonge and McManus, 1989), stress management (e.g. Michie and Sandhu, 1994), and coping skills (Ptacek *et al.*, 1994).

THREE STUDIES OF STUDENT STRESS

In this section, three studies are examined in detail which have looked at stress and coping in student health and social care professionals.

Stress in clinical psychology trainees (Cushway, 1992)

Delia Cushway conducted a postal survey of stress and coping in 287 clinical psychology trainees (response rate = 76 per cent). The average age of her sample was 27.4, 45 per cent were married or cohabiting, 78 per cent were funded on clinical psychology probationer grades, 13 per cent were on bursaries, and 9 per cent were self-funded. Stress was assessed on Goldberg's General Health Questionnaire

(Goldberg and Williams, 1988), and coping on the Health and Daily Living Schedule Adult Form B (Moos *et al.*, 1984). Clinical psychology trainees were found to have a 59 per cent caseness rate on the GHQ-28. The most frequently reported stressors were poor supervision (37 per cent), travelling (23 per cent), deadlines (22 per cent), finance (19 per cent), and moving house (19 per cent). The most frequent coping strategies were talking to other trainees (51 per cent), reducing tension through exercise (38 per cent), talking to friends (30 per cent), talking to your partner (29 per cent), and talking to your supervisor (25 per cent). Cushway also asked trainees how their training could be made less stressful. Their suggestions were :

(1) More support from course organizers and supervisors – 60 per cent.
(2) Improve course structure and organization – 39 per cent.
(3) Fewer work demands and more study time – 32 per cent.
(4) Individual therapy or personal tutor support – 29 per cent.
(5) More communication and information – 26 per cent.

Stress among student nurses (Rhead, 1995)

Rhead studied stress in two distinct groups of student nurses. Half were studying for their Registered General Nurse qualification, and the other half for the Diploma in Higher Education in Nursing. He developed a 32 item questionnaire, 16 items of which were taken from the Nurse Stress Scale (Grey-Toft and Anderson, 1981), and the other 16 items from a pilot study identifying academic stressors. Hence his measure assessed both clinical and academic work stressors. He found that RGN nursing students had significantly lower total stress scores and were most stressed by the clinical aspects of their training. By contrast Dip. HE nurses were equally stressed by the academic and clinical aspects of their training. The study raises a very important issue. It is that student health and social care professionals experience both academic and clinical pressures, unlike non-vocational student groups. The final study takes this issue a bit further.

Stress amongst three student groups (Tobin and Carson, 1994)

In this study, psychology undergraduate students ($n = 69$) were compared with social work ($n = 50$) and postgraduate certificate in education students ($n = 33$). All groups completed a demographic questionnaire, the Rosenberg Self-Esteem Scale (Rosenberg, 1965), the GHQ-28, and for the social work and PGCE students the Maslach Burnout Inventory (Maslach and Jackson, 1986). Psychology students averaged 5.48 on the GHQ-28, social work students 8.44, and PGCE students 11.64. Caseness rates were 42 per cent, 64 per cent, and 91 per cent, respectively. While Cushway (1992) was surprised to find that clinical psychology trainees had a caseness score of 59 per cent, social work and PGCE students in this study exceeded her scores. Interestingly, PGCE training combines both academic teaching and practical experience of teaching in schools. Hence it is similar to the training of health and social care professionals, which also has academic and clinical aspects, but is even more stressful!

The findings from two recent empirical studies conducted by the authors are presented next; these looked at stress in student nurses and student social workers.

STUDY 1. STRESS, COPING AND BURNOUT IN PRE-REGISTRATION AND POST-REGISTRATION NURSING STUDENTS

Methods

Procedure

Four self-report questionnaires were administered to all nursing students in a College of Health Care Studies by their tutors. Response rates were consequently very high (80 to 100 per cent of all students on each course). As sampling was conducted over a four-week period only, students not in college during this period were not surveyed. (Further details of this study are provided in Gunnoo, 1996.)

Measures

(1) Demographic Questionnaire
A 23 item questionnaire based on the work of Carson and his colleagues (Brown and Leary, 1995). This asked respondents about their age, sex, marital status, etc.

(2) Maslach Burnout Inventory
This is the most widely used measure of occupational burnout syndrome. It comprises three independent subscales: emotional exhaustion, depersonalization, and personal accomplishment. Scores are obtained for each subscale. In addition scores are categorised as high, moderate, or low in burnout, according to norms provided in the manual (Maslach and Jackson, 1986). It has 22 items.

(3) General Health Questionnaire (GHQ-28)
This is another widely used research measure. It assesses level of psychological distress (Goldberg and Williams, 1988). A total score is obtained as well as a 'caseness' rating. This last is a score of 5 or more on the 28 item form.

(4) The Cooper Coping Skills Scale
Another 28 item questionnaire, this assesses the extent to which participants use different coping strategies. There are six subscales : social support, task strategies, logic, home and work, time management, and involvement (Cooper, Sloan and Williams, 1988).

Sample

There were 183 pre-registration students, of whom 28 were completing the traditional RGN/RMN programmes, while the remainder were studying for the Diploma in Higher Education in Nursing (Project 2000). Thirty-seven were male and 146 were female. There were 269 students in the post-registration sample, comprising Enrolled Nurse conversion students, midwifery students, and other qualified nurses doing specialist English National Board courses. This sample comprised 24 men and 245 women. The samples differed significantly in the proportions of male and female students ($\chi^2 = 11.90$, d.f. = 1, $p < 0.001$). The mean age of the pre-registration students was 24.31 (standard deviation = 5.53), and for the post-registration students was 35.90 (s.d. = 8.18). This difference was also significant (Mann–Whitney $U = 5024$, $z = -13.9923$, $p < 0.0001$).

Results

(1) Findings from the Demographic Questionnaire
Some 5 per cent of pre-registration students had no sickness absence in the previous 12 months, compared with 35 per cent of post-registration students. However, more pre-registration students took more than eight days sickness absence: 23 per cent in comparison to 16 per cent for post-registration students. There were no significant differences in smoking rates: some 22 per cent of pre-registration students smoked more than 11 cigarettes per day, in contrast to 17 per cent of post-registration students. There were, however, significant differences in levels of alcohol consumption. Fewer pre-registration students were teetotal, 8 per cent versus 19 per cent, and of the regular drinkers in the sample, 18 per cent of pre-registration students consumed alcohol daily, compared to only 5 per cent of the post-registration nurses. There were also differences in job security. While 49 per cent of the pre-registration students felt they had job security, 65 per cent of the post-registration students felt secure in their jobs ($\chi^2 = 11.11$, d.f. = 1, $p < 0.001$). Finally, when asked, 'If you were finding it difficult to cope with your job who would you turn to?' pre-registration students were more likely to turn to their tutors (37 per cent), whereas post-registration students were inclined to turn to their friends (36 per cent) or colleagues (38 per cent).

(2) Maslach Burnout Inventory
Mean scores for emotional exhaustion were 16.38 for pre-registration students and 18.66 for post-registration students. So, while qualified staff reported being more emotionally drained by their jobs, these differences were not significant. Qualified staff had higher depersonalisation scores, 5.72 versus 5.28, but scored higher on personal accomplishment, 33.84 versus 32.87. There were no significant differences in the proportion of each student group falling into the high burnout category.

(3)   The General Health Questionnaire

The average GHQ total score for pre-registration students was 3.98 (s.d. = 5.11), and for post-registration students 3.38 (4.82). These differences were not significant. There were, however, significant differences in the 'caseness' rates. Some 36 per cent of pre-registration nurses scored above the criterion for caseness, in contrast to 26 per cent of post-registration nurses (χ^2 = 4.69, d.f. = 1, $p < 0.05$).

(4) The Cooper Coping Skills Scale

Scores for both groups on each subscale were as follows: social support 18.58 versus 18.63; task strategies 28.79 versus 29.25; logic 12.51 versus 12.89; home and work 17.67 versus 17.64; time 15.12 versus 15.89; involvement 25.35 versus 25.91; total coping skills 117.98 versus 120.24. Post-registration students tended to use more coping strategies overall, but the only significant difference was in the use of time management (Mann–Whitney U = 18987.5, $z = -3.2101$, $p < 0.01$).

Summary

There were surprisingly few significant differences in stress, coping and burnout in pre-registration and post-registration nurses. The main demographic differences were that pre-registration students were more likely to be regular drinkers, and also had a lower sense of job security. They scored higher on the GHQ and were more likely to be seen as 'cases'. It is possible that if a specific measure of occupational stress had been utilised in the study, such as the Harris Nurse Stress Index (Harris, 1989), then greater differences might have been apparent between the samples. Equally, a measure enabling the separation of the stress caused by academic and clinical demands for the two groups would have been helpful.

STUDY 2. STRESS, BURNOUT, AND ORGANIZATIONAL COMMITMENT AMONG STUDENT SOCIAL WORKERS

Methods

Procedure

Four self-report questionnaires were sent to student social workers from 11 different colleges. Some 652 sets of questionnaires were distributed, of which 245 (37.6 per cent) were returned. (A fuller account of this work is given in Tobin, 1995.)

Measures

(1) Demographic Questionnaire

This was an 18 item measure devised by the researchers. It covered a range of demographic details such as age, sex, marital status, etc.

(2) Maslach Burnout Questionnaire
This is described in the first study.

(3) General Health Questionnaire
Again this is described earlier.

(4) Organizational Commitment Questionnaire
Seven items from the original measure were used (Porter and Smith, 1970). This poses statements like, 'I talk up this organisation to my friends as a great organisation to work for.' Items are scored on a seven-point scale, ranging from 'strongly disagree', to 'strongly agree'.

Results

(1) Demographic Questionnaire
Females represented 77 per cent of the sample. The average age was 34 (s.d. = 7.88), 31 per cent were single, 47 per cent had children, and 80 per cent were white. Some 44 per cent had a degree.

(2) Maslach Burnout Inventory
The average scores on each subscale were as follows: emotional exhaustion = 22.55 (s.d. = 10.41), depersonalization = 6.8 (s.d. = 4.87) and personal accomplishment = 35.66 (s.d. = 5.92). Proportions of social work students falling into the high burnout categories were as follows: emotional exhaustion = 33 per cent, depersonalization = 13 per cent, and personal accomplishment = 26 per cent. In comparison with studies of other professional groups, these scores are quite high. In a table of professional scores on this scale (Leiter and Harvie, 1996), these students would have finished 4/19 on emotional exhaustion, 8/19 on depersonalization, and third from bottom on personal accomplishment.

(3) General Health Questionnaire (GHQ-28)
Average total GHQ score for this sample of social work students was 8.96 (s.d. = 7.4). The percentage caseness figure was 64 per cent. These scores are exceptionally high and well above scores for other professional groups.

(4) Organizational Commitment Questionnaire
The average score was 4.01 (s.d. = 1.44). There were few differences on this measure for any of the demographic variables. Scores were not affected by sex, age, marital status, etc.

(5) Effects of social work course type on stress and burnout
Of the sample, 154 were on diploma courses, with 85 doing either degree or postgraduate courses in social work. The samples differed significantly on age, diploma students being older, mean = 35.94, versus 31.15 for degree students.

Diploma students have an average GHQ score = 8.61 in contrast to 9.60 for degree students. This was not significant. The groups did, however, differ significantly in their Maslach scores. On emotional exhaustion, diploma students averaged 21.08 (s.d. = 10.12), degree students = 25.08 (s.d. = 10.33), (Mann–Whitney $U = 4600$, $z = -3.0854$, $p < 0.01$). Degree students are therefore more emotionally drained by their work. On depersonalization, diploma students averaged 6.17 (s.d. = 5.13), with degree students scoring 7.89 (s.d. = 5.13) (Mann–Whitney $U = 4835$, $z = 22.6040$, $p < 0.01$). Degree students are therefore less able to feel positively towards their clients. Finally on the Maslach Personal Accomplishment scale, diploma students averaged 36.36 (s.d. = 5.98), degree students = 34.46 (s.d. = 5.67) (Mann–Whitney $U = 4972.5$, $z = -2.3168$, $p < 0.05$). Diploma students feel more effective in their role.

Summary

The most striking finding to emerge from this study is the high level of stress and burnout seen in social work students. The caseness figure obtained, 64 per cent, is one of the highest of any of the professional groups yet studied. It also replicates exactly the finding of Tobin and Carson (1994), with a smaller sample of students. Equally, social work students were found to have higher levels of burnout than many professional groups previously researched. Higher levels of burnout were found in those students doing degrees than in diploma students. Adopting a more qualitative approach would again have helped determine to what extent social work students are stressed more by academic or by clinical concerns. While social work has been described as a stressful profession (Health Education Authority, 1988), it would appear that social workers experience significant levels of stress and burnout even during their training.

COMPARING NURSING AND SOCIAL WORK STUDENTS

The fact that the two studies described above used some of the same measures means that the results for the two student groups can be compared. Table 3.1 shows how social work students score more than twice as highly on the General Health Questionnaire. Indeed their scores are almost as high as for clinical samples (Carson and Brewerton, 1991). Again, caseness figures for social work students

Table 3.1 General Health Questionnaire scores

| | Nursing students | | Social work students | |
	Pre-registration	Post-registration	Diploma	Degree
Average scores	3.98 (5.11)	3.38 (4.82)	8.61 (7.24)	9.60 (7.58)
Caseness figure (%)	36	26	62	67

Standard deviations are in parentheses.

Table 3.2 Maslach Burnout Inventory Scores.

	Nursing students		Social work students	
	Pre-registration	Post-registration	Diploma	Degree
Emotional exhaustion	16.38	18.66	21.08	25.08
Depersonalization	5.28	5.72	6.17	7.89
Personal accomplishment	32.87	33.84	36.36	34.46

are also much higher, almost twice those of nursing students. Levels of psychological distress, as measured by the GHQ, are therefore considerably higher in social work students than in nursing students.

It was a similar picture for the Maslach Burnout Inventory (see Table 3.2). Social work students were more emotionally drained by their work than nursing students. Equally, they had much higher scores on depersonalization burnout. They have more cynical attitudes towards their clients. On a slightly more positive note, the social work students perceived themselves to be more effective in their role, having higher scores on personal accomplishment than had nursing students.

CONCLUSIONS

This chapter began with the speculation that training to become a health or social care professional might be a stressful process. The research literature on stress for various student groups was reviewed. Data were then presented from two separate studies that looked at stress and burnout in nursing and social work students. The study of nurses suggested that pre-registration nursing students were under slightly more stress than post-registration students. The second study demonstrated that student social workers were more than twice as stressed as nursing students according to the General Health Questionnaire. Why is the process of training to be a social worker so much more stressful than training to be a nurse? It is impossible to answer this question adequately from the present studies. Instead a more qualitative approach to discovering reasons for stress levels in the relative student groups is required. This would necessitate conducting individual interviews and focus groups with both groups of students. It may also be the case that the two professions recruit different types of student. Research on other student populations suggests that academic pressures are a major source of stress. This issue needs to be carefully addressed in future studies. While the cross-sectional research of Tobin and Carson (1994) suggests that student social workers may have more stress-prone personalities, this issue can only really be resolved by longitudinal studies. Such work would aim to measure stress levels at intake and after specified periods during the training process – before it could be stated definitively that each profession has a different stress profile.

It may, however, be of little consolation to social work students to discover that they may be under twice the stress of nursing students during their training. What they will want to know is: what can be done to reduce stress levels? This same issue has been preoccupying researchers working with medical students. These workers have postulated that if medical students can be taught to recognize personal stress reactions and to develop adaptive coping mechanisms, then they may not experience so much stress when they are qualified (Coombes, Perell and Ruckh, 1990; Michie and Sandhu, 1994). The research presented in this chapter suggests that there may be an urgent need to introduce similar stress management programmes for social work students.

REFERENCES

Bramness, J. Fixdal, T. and Vaglum, P. (1991) Effect of medical school stress on the mental health of medical students in early and late clinical curriculum. *Acta Psychiatrica Scandanavica*, **84** (4), 340–5.

Brown, D. and Leary, J. (1995) Findings from the Claybury study for community psychiatric nurses, in *Stress and Coping in Mental Health Nursing,* (eds J. Carson, L. Fagin, and S. Ritter), Chapman and Hall, London.

Carson, J. and Brewerton, T. (1991) Out of the clinic into the classroom. *Adults Learning*, **2** (9), 256–7.

Cheng, D. Leong, F. and Geist, R. (1993) Cultural differences between Asian and Caucasian American college students. *Journal of Multicultural Counselling and Development*, **21** (3), 182–90.

Coombes, R. Perell, K. and Ruckh, J. (1990) Primary prevention of emotional impairment among medical trainees. *Academic Medicine*, **65** (9), 576–81.

Cooper, C., Sloan, S. and Williams, S. (1988) *Occupational Stress Indicator Management Guide*, NFER–Nelson, Windsor.

Cushway, D. (1992) Stress in clinical psychology trainees. *British Journal of Clinical Psychology*, **31**, 169–79.

Everly, J., Poff, D., Lamport, N. *et al.* (1994) Perceived stressors and coping strategies of occupational therapy students. *American Journal of Occupational Therapy*, **48** (11), 1022–8.

Gadzella, B. (1994) Student Life Stress Inventory: identification of and reactions to stressors. *Psychological Reports*, **74** (2), 395–402.

Goldberg, D. and Williams, P. (1988) *A User's Guide to the General Health Questionnaire*. NFER–Nelson, Windsor.

Grey-Toft, P. and Anderson, J. (1981) The Nursing Stress Scale: development of an instrument. *Journal of Behavioural Assessment*, **3**, 11–23.

Gunnoo, V. (1996) Stress, coping and burnout in pre- and post-registration nursing students. Thesis submitted for MSc in Mental Health Interventions. Middlesex University.

Harris, P. (1989) The Nurse Stress Index. *Work and Stress*, **3**, 335–46.

Health Education Authority (1988) *Stress in the Public Sector: Nurses, Police, Social Workers and Teachers*, Health Education Authority, London.

Kohn, P. and Gurevich, M. (1993) On the adequacy of the indirect method of measuring the primary appraisal of hassles based stress. *Personality and Individual Differences*, **14** (5), 679–84.

Leiter, M. and Harvie, P. (1996) Burnout among mental health workers: a review and research agenda. *International Journal of Social Psychiatry*, **42** (2) 90–101.

Lindop, E. (1989) Individual stress and its relationship to termination of nurse training. *Nurse Education Today*, **9** (3), 172–9.

Maslach, C. and Jackson, S. (1986) *Maslach Burnout Inventory*. Consulting Psychologists Press, California.

Michie, S. and Sandhu, S. (1994) Stress management for clinical medical students. *Medical Education*, **28** (6), 528–33.

Moos, R. Cronkite, R. Billings, A. and Finney, J. (1984) *Health and Daily Form Manual*. Social Ecology Laboratory, Stanford University, Palo Alto.

Mosley, T., Perrin, S. Neral, S. *et al.*, (1994) Stress, coping and well-being among third year medical students. *Academic Medicine*, **69** (9), 765–7.

Porter, L. and Smith, R. (1970) The etiology of organizational commitment. University of California, unpublished paper.

Ptacek, J., Smith, R., Espe, K. and Rafferty, B. (1994) Limited correspondence between daily coping reports and retrospective coping recall. *Psychological Assessment*, **6** (1,) 41–9.

Ramanaidu, S. (1991) A comparison of stresses experienced by home and overseas students of radiography. *Radiography Today*, **57** (645), 18–27.

Rhead, M. (1995) Stress among student nurses: is it practical or academic? *Journal of Clinical Nursing*, **4**, 369–76.

Rocha-Singh, I. (1994) Perceived stress among graduate students : development and validation of the Graduate Stress Inventory. *Educational and Psychological Measurement*, **54** (3), 714–27.

Rosenberg, M. (1965) *Society and the Adolescent Self-Image*. Princeton University Press, Princeton.

Sandhu, D. (1994) An examination of the psychological needs of international students : implications for counselling and psychotherapy. *International Journal for the Advancement of Counselling*, **17** (4), 229–39.

Scullion, P. (1994) Identification of stressors associated with student nurses in an accident and emergency department and comparison of stress levels. *Accident and Emergency Nursing*, **2** (2), 79–86.

Solberg, V., Hale, J., Vilarreal, P. and Kavanagh, J. (1993) Development of the College Stress Inventory for use with Hispanic populations: a confirmatory factor analytic study. *Hispanic Journal of Behavioural Sciences*, **15** (4), 490–7.

Tobin, P. J. (1995) Professional training, stress, burnout and organisational committment. Thesis submitted for MSc in Occupational and Organisational Psychology. University of East London.

Tobin, P. J. and Carson, J. (1994) Stress and the student social worker. *Social Work and Social Sciences Review*, **5** (3), 246–55.

Tooth, D., Tonge, K. and McManus, I. (1989) Anxiety and study methods in preclinical students: causal relation to examination performance. *Medical Education*, **23** (5), 416–21.

Um, M. and Brown-Standrige, M. (1993) Discovering organisational rules that contribute to student stress in social work field placements. *Journal of Applied Social Sciences*, **17** (2), 157–77.

4	# Organizations in the mind: the interaction of organizational and intrapsychic perspectives

Christopher Rance

INTRODUCTION

In my role as management consultant, I have, over the years, come to know many very different organizations, more than would have been possible in a more traditional career development path. I have been impressed how many people I met who were unhappy in their work most of the time. Under stress people will say, 'surely there are other places where people work in harmony, acknowledge each other's valuable contribution to the task at hand. Almost any other place would appreciate my contribution/talents/brilliant ideas better than this one.' Those who are long-term members of a particular organization tend to think that the awfulness of their workplace is unique to their own particular situation; they find it difficult even to entertain the idea that work-related stress is a common experience of the human condition.

In my experience, however, although each workplace has its particular characteristics and situations which can contribute to stress in its members, I find that debilitating stress is often experienced when these characteristics cannot really be held to be the principal cause.

I have found that the extent to which the experience of work is seen as rewarding and fulfilling appears to be largely independent of the specifics of the workplace and is drawn from the internal mental resources and social perspectives of the individuals concerned. It seems that unhappiness, stress, and anger are as independent of the external specifics of a given working environment as are job fulfilment and job satisfaction. The same work experience can produce extreme anger and anxiety in one person and amused tolerance in another. A simple example of this occurred recently in a local District General Hospital where bright new road signs appeared one day pointing to the 'Physiotherapy Department', which, when carefully followed, led to the doors of the Psychotherapy Department, now relabelled Physiotherapy. The depth of the feelings of threat experienced by some of the staff involved was impressive but clearly disproportionate to the error.

I have come to the conclusion that we are all to a large degree, as individuals, not so much passive victims of the stresses and strains of a hostile organization and its machinations 'out there', but are creative participants in the organization, and that many of the perceived stresses and anxieties, and their intensity, find their source in our own intrapsychic perspectives and the interpsychic interactions and communications we have with our work colleagues.

I would like to describe here a paradigm of the workplace in which the individual and the work group, the interactions between myself and others, can be viewed as different perspectives of the same psychic reality. This paradigm is based on the view that all meaning is contained in interpersonal communication and that it is in communication that we can access the reality of our mental world and that of others. It can help to make sense of our experience of the workplace that Freud (1930, p. 264) made the following observation about this so important and so disliked an experience:

> No other technique for the conduct of life attaches the individual so firmly to reality as laying emphasis on work; for his work at least gives him a secure place in a portion of reality, in the human community. ... And yet, as a path to happiness, work is not highly prized by men. They do not strive after it as they do after other possibilities of satisfaction. The great majority of people only work under the stress of necessity, and this natural human aversion to work raises most difficult social problems.

There are three key concepts of the development of personality which contribute to our understanding of our relationships with people and the external world. They are the three strands of developmental theory which constitute the group analytic paradigm and are drawn from social psychology, psychoanalysis, and systems theory. I will then apply them to the concepts of organization, management, and work group, which together constitute organizational group analysis.

THE SOCIAL ORIGINS OF PERSONALITY

The strand of social psychology, which is particularly relevant in this context, owes its origins to the work of George Herbert Mead as developed by the sociologist Norbert Elias at Leicester and Frankfurt Universities. Elias explored (1991, p. 60) the notions of the social origins of personality and developed the concept of the 'Society of Individuals', and the gestalt of the We–I, where the individual mental process and the interpersonal process are seen as being formally part of the same mental process.

What are often conceptually separated as two different substances or two different strata within the human being, his 'individuality' and his 'social conditioning', are in fact nothing other than two different functions of people in their relations to each other, one of which cannot exist without the other. They are terms for the specific activity of the individual in relation to his fellows, and for his capacity to be influenced and shaped by their activity; for the dependence of others on him and his dependence on others, expressions for his function as both *die* and *coin*.

The strength of this idea is that it is not a social metaphor for personal development but a key analogy. By 'analogy' I mean a circumstance where two or more things, existing separately, share the same form. In this case there is a formal unity between the process in the mind of the individual and the social communication in the group matrix. The group comes into existence by virtue of the communication between individuals who have been ontologically formed in a social context. The 'I' that can talk about the 'me' is the 'I' that has first learnt about objects of knowledge in social interaction with others and only later about the 'me' as an object of knowledge to which the 'I' as knower can refer. The individual mental processes are therefore a formal representation of the group processes and vice versa in continuous interchange. In the group context we can see the individuals and the group as single analogously figured gestalts of foreground and background in continual interchange.

As Ian Burkitt (1991, p. 188) summarises in his commentary on Norbert Elias:

... our personalities are formed within social structures, the dynamics of which are not totally revealed to our consciousness. Also the repressed elements of our personalities are formed in the same social processes as those elements of which we are consciously aware.

PSYCHOANALYSIS AND THE UNCONSCIOUS

An important part of the social interaction through which we come to know ourselves in relation to others happens without conscious awareness. Psychoanalytic theory offers a valuable perspective on the development of the person in relation to others from the earliest preverbal stages of mental life. It holds that these early mental phenomena underpin the emotional development of the individual and unconsciously permeate styles of perception and relating throughout life. An excellent introduction to these ideas is to be found in the introduction to psychoanalysis by Robert Caper (1988).

Central to psychoanalysis is the idea that anxiety arises in relation to both real and imagined dangers and that a new-born infant is not well equipped to cope with emotional states that might later be recognized as fear or frustration or anxiety. The child is born dependent on its mother, father, and other adult care givers to make sense of its emotional states and to take appropriate action to allay its fears.

Since this process never happens perfectly the child also develops defence. against anxiety. Early defences have a special quality of omnipotence and involve major distortions in the perception of self and of external reality. The most extreme forms of defence involve an attack on the mind itself and on its capacity to perceive reality. With increasing maturity the distortions of perception become more circumscribed although there is always an element of denial of that aspect of reality which is too painful or anxiety provoking to bear. Early defences are organized around the phenomena of splitting, projection, and identification – complex unconscious processes which distort the nature of the other as perceived in external reality and of the self experienced subjectively. This occurs through a concrete unconscious fantasy of forceful projection into the other of split-off and disowned aspects of the self in relation to the other. For example, an experience of frustration in relation to the other's unavailability may be experienced as a hostile exclusion of one's self by the other. The anger at being thwarted is unconsciously transferred to the other, thus transforming a simple fact into a deliberate persecutory act.

As a general rule the more stressed a person is, the more they will tend to resort to earlier defences, in other words the more prone they will be to misinterpret reality in terms of early emotional prototypes. In the example above the other's unavailability was experienced more as a nursing infant might feel if when he cried with hunger and his mother did not come.

A less stressed individual or the same person in a less stressed state is able to deal with these prototypical anxieties and hurts more rationally. 'Well I know that she asked me to phone between 11.00 and 11.30 a.m. but she has probably been delayed/called to deal with an emergency etc.' If, however, this was the twentieth time something similar had happened we might suspect the caller to be defending himself by rationalizing against the realization that she was avoiding him.

In any interpersonal context each individual's inner world (the sum of fantasy, anxiety, and defence in relation to previous significant others) will inevitably impinge to a degree on their capacity to perceive and interpret another's intentions accurately. This means that all social interaction is permeated to a degree by transference and counter-transference phenomena. 'Transference' means relating to the unavailable other as if she were (in our example above) the unavailable mother of one's infancy. With counter-transference the feelings are stirred up in the other (often unconsciously) of having such an attribution visited upon them. In our example the absent person might actually react with hostility to too forceful a reproach about her unavailability. Larry Hirschhorn (1988) takes these ideas further with his exploration of the ideas of work as a reparative process of 'making it better' with those we have hated in the past for 'not being there'.

It is easy to see how such unconscious processes will inevitably impinge on experiences in the workplace. It is crucial in terms of the social origins of our personality as described by Elias that we distinguish in the one mental relational process those elements that originate in our own past experiences and our own unconscious, and those that may not.

SYSTEMS THEORY AND THE EMERGENT PROPERTIES OF SYSTEMS

The third perspective of the psychosocial relationship between the individual and the group, the whole and the part, is drawn from general systems theory. Both the human mind and the organization are seen metaphorically as a system. From the Solar System to the bee hive, from economics to atomic physics, the natural world and the way it is organized can be described in terms of systems. The system is a metaphor for the relationship between the individual and the group which is all the more powerful because we *are* systems at both the individual and the group level.

A system, viewed structurally, is a divisible whole; viewed functionally, it is an indivisible whole, since its essential properties are a function of the organization of the parts and are lost by dismantling it. (Consider a clock.) The system is a complex of elements or components directly or indirectly related in a causal network, such that each component is related to at least some others in a more or less stable way within any particular period of time. The structure of the system at any particular time is determined by the particular kinds of more or less stable interrelationships of the components that become established at that time. The system, with its structure and organization, is a whole with continuity in time and with a boundary in actual or, for our argument, conceptual space.

A closed system manifests the second law of thermodynamics: it reaches equilibrium and thereafter can do no more work and entropy is maximal; this is what Freud redefined in psychological terms as the death instinct. An open system exchanges energy, materials, and signals with its environment and, by processing its inputs in ways that are constantly changing to match its environment, produces output that is appropriate to that environment. It is important to ascertain in what ways the individual, the group, and the organization in the mind are closed or open systems. An individual, a group, or an organization in the mind which is closed down by anxiety is a closed system and can do no more work.

In systemic terms, the mind can be seen as an emergent property of the central nervous system. In the same way the awareness of the mental construct of 'organization' can be seen as an emergent property of the social interaction of the participating collaborators.

General systems theory is by itself an 'empty' theory, that is, it has form but no intrinsic content. In conjunction with the sociological analogy of mental process, the insights of psychoanalysis and the unconscious, it is very useful in formalizing our understanding of organizations and in proposing an ongoing process of change.

To these three psychological perspectives (which are really three ways of looking at the same developmental psychological processes) I would like to add three key mental constructs that are closely related ways in which we conceptualize our interpersonal learning experiences.

ORGANIZATION

We all belong to many very different organizations but we firstly think of the one where we most express our hopes and ambitions – the workplace. Organization is primarily a mental construct, rather like 'society', 'traffic', or the 'corporate entity' of company law, which only exist as entities in the minds of those participating in them. A corporate entity is described as immortal and immaterial and is manifested by 'its members for the time being'. The concept of 'mind' itself is a mental construct derived, as we have seen, from social interaction. An organization in this sense is formed by the interaction of all its members trying to make sense of where they find themselves in a particular context. It is the expression of a network of relationships, as entertained in the minds of those concerned, unlike the idea of 'institution' which consists of the articles of association, the bricks and mortar, and the bank balances with which the organization functions, and which is often 'owned' by someone quite other than the work force. I do not mind if the terms are reversed, so long as the distinction is clear, although 'organization' etymologically suggests the dynamic process and 'institution' the static one.

The idea of 'organization' as a mental construct is well described by Argyris and Schön (1980, p. 131):

> Each member of the organisation constructs his or her own representation, or image, of the theory-in-use [actual behaviour] of the whole. That picture is always incomplete. The organisation members strive continually to complete it, and to understand themselves in the context of the organisation. They try to describe themselves and their own performance in so far as they interact with others. As conditions change, they test and modify that description. Moreover, others are continually engaged in similar enquiry. It is this continual, concerted meshing, of one's activities in the context of collective interaction, which constitutes an organisation's knowledge of its theory in use.

We can all usefully work with organizational metaphors such as learning systems, hierarchies, organisms, systems, brains, cultures, implicate/explicate orders, psychoanalytic defences, power structures, and anthropological parallels, as well described by Gareth Morgan (1986). However, the fact that there are so many popular metaphors confirms that 'organization' is an elusive mental construct. It is often important to clarify which mental model someone is using when describing an organization 'in the mind' if one is not to be misled by the inherent weaknesses of any particular model. The default model in our society is probably that of hierarchy, which is daily re-enforced by pyramidal organization charts. Whichever model one uses, it can only be actualized through the process of communication between its members. The mode of communication defined by the default model is an authoritarian one.

MANAGEMENT

In a similar way 'management' is a related mental construct. Our definitions of 'management', and the ways in which we will try to engage in appropriate communication with others at work to exercise it as a role, differ greatly, depending on the image of organization in the mind to which we subscribe. Problems immediately arise if different models are at play in the same workplace. As Peter Senge, (1990, p. 185) observes, in his discussion on the nature of management:

> the impact of mental models on managers' understanding is profound – most report that they see for the first time in their life that all we ever have are assumptions, never 'truths', that we always see the world through our mental models and that mental models are always incomplete and in Western culture, chronically non-systemic.

As a mental construct 'management' can be seen, irrespective of model, as primarily the perception of the network of relationships in the workplace as viewed by each individual. It can be defined as the management of one's self in the presence of others, in the context of a collaborative task. It is how I see myself in relation to others, partly in response to how I perceive them, individually and/or collectively, viewing me, and partly driven by my own expectations. Management is only secondarily the management of the work group's 'self' in the presence of other work groups. Finally it can be seen as the management of the enterprise as a whole in the socioeconomic context in which it operates. The task of designated 'management' as 'other' is essentially to facilitate this process, starting at the personal one, and initially by example. Just as management is primarily a process of self-realization, it is also, at the level of the work group and beyond, a process of social self-realization and discovery.

Just as the concrete correlates of organization in the mind are in the institution, so the concrete correlates of management are the institutional structures: the necessary forms of leadership, power and authority, responsibility, accountability, rules and regulations, and financial constraints. These are necessary for the completion of the tasks of the institution but their meaning is to be found in our own and others' mental constructs, largely unrelated to the specific institutional structures.

WORK GROUP

A 'work group' can be defined as a collection of people who collaborate together, each with a separate, if not different, role, for the completion of a set range of tasks. It is a mental construct of relationship that exists in our heads irrespective of whether we are actually at work. When we talk about work groups we are often really referring to specific daily meetings of the team. These sessions, however, only have the task of facilitating communication between its members; the actual numbers who attend do not qualitatively change the nature of the group.

As Wilfred Bion (1961, p. 131) observed, a group is independent of time and space (being as it is, a mental construct) and only meets in a particular place at a particular time for convenience:

> In his Group Psychology and the Analysis of the Ego, Freud opens his discussion by pointing out that individual and group psychology cannot be absolutely differentiated because the psychology of the individual is itself a function of the individual's relationship to an other person or object. He objects (p. 3) that it is difficult to attribute to the factor of number a significance so great as to make it capable by itself of moving in over mental life a new instinct that is not otherwise brought into play. In my view, no new instinct is brought into play, it is always in play. ... It is necessary for a group to meet in a room because the conditions for study can be provided only in that way.

The specific meetings of the team have no independent existence other than a spaciotemporal representation of the work group, which like the organization has its primary existence in the mind of the participants. The meetings influence the group in so far as they afford an opportunity for each member of the team present to influence, through communication, other members' mental constructs of the team and each member's role in it. To give a specific meeting (or a team's specific daily attendance) a separate reality is to attribute too much significance to number. The primary reality of the work group is a psychological rather than a physical presence. It is also analogous in terms of communication with both the mental constructs of 'management' and 'organization' as described above.

The concrete correlates to the mental constructs of the work group are the tasks, designated roles, and interdisciplinary arrangements within the work group. It is impressive how many people imagine that the utilization of the skills of individuals in the work group and their effectiveness are specific to the nature of the task in hand rather than to the psychological perspectives and mental constructs of the group members in interaction with one another. I have found that people will often reject an assertion from a consultant that the same jobs can be done just as well in totally different ways, that they can be done with different skill mixes, and that the way things are done in a particular situation is as much an expression of the interpsychic life of the work group as it is of the realities of the tasks at hand.

THE GROUP ANALYTIC PARADIGM AND DIALOGUE

How can we then use these psychosocial theories and organizational mental constructs in a coherent paradigm to help us manage in the institutions in which we find ourselves? More accurately, how can we understand the organizations that we encounter daily in our minds, and the many overlapping organizations that constitute our experience of the workplace? How can we minimize realistic stresses, optimally function in our work roles, facilitate task achievement, and make personal fulfilment a reality for both ourselves and others? What can we do on our own behalf and what can we, in as much as we have a responsibility for promoting the productive collaboration of others, actually do to make unconscious fears and stresses conscious and therefore less absolute in their power to control and to reduce collaborative effectiveness?

In particular, do we attend to the organization, to the management, to the work groups, or to individuals? What is the best level of focus? The answer is that they are all formally similar and the individual's self-awareness is the window on to the processes of the group. As S.H. Foulkes (1990, p. 223) observed,

> Psychology is [thus] neither 'individual' or 'group'; except by abstraction. We cannot speak about the individual without reference to the group nor about a human group that does not consist of individuals. Both are therefore abstractions as far as the psychology of the total person is concerned. We can focus on the group as a whole or on any one individual or individuals in their specific interactions; all that happens is meaningful from any point of view and all the meanings dovetail.

In maintaining that the reality of the workplace is experienced in our emotional perceptions and their modification in light of current experience, we necessarily start with ourselves and our own internal world. We will find we are much more empowered by this than if we have to rely on understanding and changing others in order to have a constructive effect on our work group.

The starting point for either work colleagues or consultants follows the tripartite psychosocial model I have described above.

(1) We can maintain that it is the responsibility of all individual members of the work group to understand at least some of the psychosocial origins of their own personalities and their impact on their current intra-group behaviour patterns. It is our responsibility to access the mental process of the group by being aware of and examining the formally self-same mental process in ourselves and taking responsibility for them rather than trying to 'understand' others in an instrumental sense. The formal similarity of the process in others will lead us to understand others only in so far as we have managed to be in touch with our own mental constructs and processes.

(2) It is the responsibility of each of us to recognize the psychoanalytically informed dimensions of this social process of group relationships, by becoming aware of our own unconscious processes, as far as is possible, by the recognition of our own defences, transferences, and counter-transferences, as they contribute to the maladaptive unconscious elements of our relationships with others. Again, the only access we have to the unconscious processes of others is in the understanding of our own counter-transferences, and not in claiming to have insights into others' mental constructs directly.

(3) It is the responsibility of each of us to learn in collaboration with others and thus, in a systemic sense, to change both the input and process of the system

by modifying our own, and therefore everyone else's, view of the organization, management, and work group (in the mind). It is our responsibility to acknowledge both our interdependence and the inescapable interactive facets of our collaboration and their effects on the outputs of the system. In other words our own ability to learn is the controlling factor and not any imagined skills of teaching.

In group analytic terms, all meaning is in the communication of individuals in creative interaction. The ability to understand and develop the organization rests with each member taking responsibility for learning about their own internal process and not in presuming, in an instrumental sense, to take responsibility for the mental processes of others. The formal process of this developmental learning, as opposed to its context or its content, is creative communication. Pat de Maré (1991, p. 64), a group analyst, called it 'dialogue':

> Dialogue is the hallmark of the human species and is an *a priori* form of currency: it is the skill that has to be learnt and used if humans are to survive the onslaughts of human mismanagement let alone Nature. People speak to each other in a creative, emerging manner. Mind does not emerge automatically: it is an outcome of a dynamic tension continuously in dialogue, a continuous miracle of psycho-genesis.

This concept has been taken up by David Böhm (1989) and Peter Senge (1990), who go on to describe 'dialogue' in terms of particle physics and organizational learning, respectively, as the promotion of learning and change by internal self-awareness and the collaborative interchange of ideas, leading to new thoughts or ideas. Dialogue in the group is a process of communal interactive learning rather than teaching, of changing oneself rather than others, and learning about the psychic realities of oneself in each new group context, rather than about defining the internal mental processes of others.

Dialogue, as the expression of the mental constructs of the participating members of a given organization (management team or work group), is the primary function of group analytic organizational understanding and intervention. It is not a simple process. It has in itself potential for stressful interaction. It can, however, be likened to the art of conversation where the skill is in creative listening not talking. The only useful outcome of a group meeting or conversation, is a new idea, not present in the minds of anyone before the meeting. To wait in a state of unknowing until the idea occurs is the experience of frustration and uncertainty. The temptation is often to foreclose the process with 'here is an idea I had earlier'.

MANAGEMENT PROCESSES: GROUP OR INDIVIDUAL?

The current vogue for shallow organizational structures with no supervisory management levels means that work groups are becoming more autonomous. This is technically quite feasible in today's computerized environment. The sociological implications will require, however, a more complex paradigm of psychosocial processes in management terms than has previously been readily available, if debilitating stresses are to be mitigated. The designated leader or management group is the facilitating role model for optimizing the communications processes only in so far as it is in their power, by learning and relearning (changing) on a daily basis, to help others to learn, relearn, and manage for themselves. It requires the acceptance that one can only have any real power over one's own internal world.

Although 'management' (like 'organization' and 'work group') is primarily an individual mental construct and personal process, there is in practice one group of people in an institution whose opinions and interpersonal mental constructs will have a disproportionately influential impact on the organization as a whole, whether for beneficial change or increasing entropy. This is the group of designated 'managers' or authority-empowered leaders. These groups can and often do affect an organization by inappropriate behaviour which leads to massive systemic failures, well documented in the management literature. Management styles under such conditions include management by patronage, by threats, witch hunting, blaming, buck passing, the divorce of authority and responsibility, opaque bureaucracy, etc. These are easily recognizable but difficult to stop once started.

There is always the tendency that under stress groups will malfunction. Mental constructs of organization, management, and work group tend to destabilize under excessive stress. Ideas are elevated to the level of idols which cannot be questioned. Corporate history is littered with patently silly ideas that seemed to otherwise sensible people to be good ideas at the time. What aberration of thought processes led the Conservative Cabinet to think the Poll Tax was a good idea? Such management group failures and reverses are well known but the power of such groups for successful development through creative dialogue has not had the same exposure.

The unsung heroes of corporate life are in fact those management groups who function well together in personal terms as well as financial ones and empower others to do the same. The only real measure of success in the human sphere is in the appropriately low level of stress to be found in the individuals who make up the organization, the management, and the work groups of a successful institution. The long-term successes of the Quaker family industrialists were based on their enlightened respect for the individual worker. Their perspectives were overtly religious rather than secularly psychological but the results were what we are all aiming at.

STRESS AS THE BAROMETER OF ORGANIZATIONAL LIFE

The group analytic 'democratization of organizational life', achieved by placing its primary reality in the minds of individuals and their mental constructs, means that the key to a fulfilling organizational life lies not in our stars but in ourselves. Freud once described the function of psychoanalysis as the conversion of the moments of hysterical suffering to those of commonplace unhappiness. The group analytic paradigm aims to have similarly modest claims. Some stress is a necessary part of all interaction, psychosocial learning, and working together, but not too much.

In systemic terms the process of increased self-awareness will result in internal mental changes in oneself, which will either systemically lead to an acceptable change in the organization and its levels of stress, an acceptable change in the individual and his or her levels of stress, or a mutually beneficial parting of the ways for both. Change depends, however, on whether the systems concerned are closed or open and available for thought.

Individuals under stress must ask themselves to what degree this stress can be understood in terms of past personal developmental experiences defining present mental constructs and relationships. They must ascertain whether the system is open to change or is closed, starting with the system of their own mental world. Many systems, both personal and organizational (in as much as one can distinguish these) are closed, ceasing to function appropriately and becoming highly stressed. Many people never learn to get on with others and eventually, without psychological help, become unemployable. Corporate entities may not die but many certainly tend towards entropy; there are very few in this country over 75 years old.

In practical terms the self-awareness of an individual's stress levels is a valuable indicator of the possibilities of internal change having an effect on the interactive reality of the organization in the mind. If changes in individual perceptions are significant enough, there might be some concrete anxiety-reducing manifestation of beneficial change in the organization; the system is changing appropriately (improving). There might, however, be no concrete manifestation of change but the individual stress levels may reduce; this might suggest that the individual perception of the organization is changing appropriately (improving).

If no beneficial changes occur and individual stresses are maintained at an unacceptably high level, then either the process of individual learning has closed down under the stress or the ideas for change have not had enough impact on others to overcome the natural entropy of the system. In either case the only way to reduce individual stress to an acceptable level may be for individuals to absent themselves from the organization by leaving the institution.

Eventually everyone leaves a closed system unless the organization, as experienced in the minds of its members, can change enough to avoid inappropriate stress. Stress levels are the barometer of the potential for change and its realization at the individual level, the group level, the management level, and the larger organizational level, which, as we have seen here, are all formally part of the same process.

REFERENCES

Argyris, C. and Schön, D. (1980) What is an organisation that it may learn? in *Organisations as Systems* (eds M. Lockett, and R. Spear), Open University Press, Milton Keynes, pp. 128–37.

Bion, W. R. (1961) *Experiences in Groups,* SSP Tavistock, London.

Böhm, D. (1989) *On Dialogue*, David Böhm Seminars, Ojai, CA.

Burkitt, I. (1991) *Social Selves: Theories of The Social Formulation of Personality,* Sage Publications, London.

Caper, R. (1988) *Immaterial Facts – Freud's Discovery of Psychic Reality and Klein's Development of His Work,* Aronson, London.

de Maré, P. (1991) Dialogue, in *Koinonia. From Hate through Dialogue to Culture in the Large Group* (eds P. de Maré *et al.*), Karnac, London, pp. 41–74.

Elias, N. (1991) *The Society of Individuals,* Basil Blackwell, Oxford.

Foulkes, S.H. (1990) The group as matrix of the individual's mental life, in *Selected Papers, Psychoanalysis and Group Analysis* (cd. E. Foulkes), Karnac, London, pp. 223–33.

Freud S. (1930) *Civilisation and Its Discontents*, The Pelican Freud Library, Volume 12, Penguin, Harmondsworth, pp. 251–340.

Hirschhorn, L. (1988) *The Workplace Within, Psychodynamics of Organisational Life,* MIT Press, London.

Morgan, G. (1986) *Images of Organisation*, Sage Publications, London.

Senge, P. M. (1990) *The Fifth Discipline – The Art and Practice of the Learning Organisation,* Doubleday, London.

Caring for health care professionals – with special reference to physicians

5

Sydney Brandon

The cobbler's children go barefoot.

Old English proverb

Freudenberger (1984) described the syndrome of 'burnout', which he believed to be particularly common among health care workers. This syndrome was said to be characterized by emotional exhaustion, depersonalization, and low productivity with feelings of low achievement.

Nurses have high rates of sickness absence, smoke more, and commit suicide more than the general population. The high rates of attrition from the nursing profession have been a matter of concern for many years (Secombe, Ball and Patch, 1993). Isabel Menzies (1960) in a classic study drew attention to the anxiety-generating structure of the nursing profession. A distinguished psychiatrist, discussing sick role behaviour in nurses, observed that the desire to nurse is often closely linked with the desire to be nursed (Roth,1960). Many trusts are introducing punitive approaches to the taking of sick leave, making staff feel like anonymous units of production. Concern over job security is increasing and more and more nurses want to leave the profession (Collee, 1993).

Health service managers have generated less sympathy but a number of recent studies have demonstrated levels of morbidity in senior managers comparable to those in senior medical staff (Caplan, 1994). The lack of security of tenure, the high expectations of themselves and their employers, and the unpopularity of many of the changes they are required to implement all contribute to the high stress levels.

A number of studies have noted an excess of health problems in most occupational groups related to medicine. Balarajan (1989) showed that for men, overall mortality as indicated by the standardized mortality rate (SMR), based on the 1971 and 1981 censuses, was significantly lower in dentists (66), doctors (69), opticians (72), and physiotherapists (79), whereas the SMRs were significantly higher among hospital porters (151), nurses (118), and ambulancemen (109). Table 5.1 shows that all groups of hospital workers other than ambulancemen had raised SMRs for suicide and cirrhosis.

It is, however, the health problems of physicians that have received the greatest attention and are now a matter of apparently increasing concern (British Medical Association, 1992, 1993). Doctors are a scarce, expensive, and valuable resource and there are not enough of them to meet identified demands. Current manpower and training requirements in the United Kingdom have resulted in reduced flexibility in employing the available pool of trained doctors.

Qualification in medicine brings automatic membership of an upper social class with expectations of good health, good income, an assured and satisfying job, and identification with a respected profession. At the same time, membership demands an acceptance of the prevailing mores of medicine. There is an ethos in medicine which carries an expectation of dedication, hard work, and long hours. Commitment to the individual patient and to the service make it difficult for the physician to abandon this care obligation because of personal ill health. The structure of the service is such that if an individual doctor is unexpectedly absent there is usually no one to provide alternative cover. Either the patient is not dealt with or colleagues must assume responsibility over and above their already full commitment. The 'Patient's Charter' requires that patients should be seen within a defined time and this adds to the problems. There is an imperative to most health problems and patients are reluctant to postpone their appointment whether it be for diagnosis or treatment. Whatever the reasons, doctors are usually reluctant to become patients. Most resort to self-diagnosis and prescription. Junior doctors are particularly prone to seek advice from their peers or from those barely senior to them. The more senior trainees and established doctors often seek help on an informal basis with consultations in the corridor or at social occasions rather than

Table 5.1 Standardized mortality rates for various occupations (men only), 1979–1983, England and Wales (from Balarajan, 1989)

Occupation	Suicide	Cirrhosis
Doctors	172	177
Dentists	222	165
Pharmacists	242	254
Nurses	201	121
Porters	184	232
Ambulance men	77	22
Orderlies	144	162
Hospital manual workers	141	159

in a clinic or surgery. Partly as a consequence of this informality and consultation without notes or systematic investigation, doctors often receive less than adequate care. Many doctors are reluctant to consult their GP, many juniors have failed to register with a doctor locally, and more senior doctors often sign on with some local doyen or one with whom they work closely and are unwilling to consult on sensitive matters. Most doctors have reservations about using their local services for reasons of confidentiality or fear of meeting patients or colleagues. The extra contractual referral (ECR) system is making it more difficult to consult outside the local facilities.

For whatever reason, doctors tend to be late in consulting on serious matters and with alcohol or other drug abuse they consult on average after more than six years of abuse (Brooke, Edwards and Taylor, 1991); for psychological distress similar reluctance and delay are evident (Vincent, 1969).

Another major factor is of course the fear of being judged unfit to practice by peers, by employers, or by the General Medical Council (GMC). Until comparatively recently the National Health Service was a monopoly employer and dismissal from an NHS post could result in virtual blacklisting. Although there are now more opportunities in private practice it is doubtful whether a doctor who has left the NHS under a cloud would be welcome in a private clinic. In the case of GPs, many will be aware of colleagues whose partnerships have been dissolved when they revealed the existence of a health problem. Many doctors who leave a general practice or hospital post because of illness become peripatetic locums – perhaps the worst situation for a person with problems of health or performance.

Although the GMC has as its primary task the protection of the public, it does attempt to deal sympathetically with doctors who are affected by illness. Through the Health Committee it is often able to deal with such problems without publicity. Despite this many doctors have an irrational fear that the GMC will intervene if they become ill, particularly if the illness is prolonged or involves mental disturbance or drugs. Even experienced doctors may believe that details of their illness will be provided to their employer or to the GMC.

The standardized mortality rate (SMR) for doctors has improved from 81 (i.e. 19 per cent better than average) in 1968 to 66 or 34 per cent better than average in 1988. There is however a down side with: SMR suicide 331; SMR cirrhosis 311; SMR accidents 180. Lung cancer deaths had declined for the profession until 1971, since when there has been a slow rise. Alcoholic cirrhosis rates, mental hospital admissions, and referrals to the GMC disciplinary committee are 5.5 times higher than the overall United Kingdom rate for Scots and nine times greater for Irish graduates. There is evidence of underreporting of suicide among doctors (Richings, Khara and McDowell, 1986) and of inadequate reporting of morbidity partly due to the fact that many fail to take or to report sick leave.

The medical profession poses particular problems, for, despite a low rate of actual sickness absence, high morbidity levels can be demonstrated at every stage of the medical career. Doctors face real difficulties in shaping their careers (Ashley-Miller and Lehmann, 1993). It is estimated that undergraduate education may cost up to £200,000 with the possibility of as much again being expended on postgraduate education and training.

Medical students show high stress levels early in their course and these seem to be independent of gender. As they progress through their clinical years to the pre-registration house officer (PRHO) posts there is evidence of a steep rise in manifestations of stress, and rates for women begin to exceed those for men. The prevalence of emotional disturbance in pre-registration housemen is reported as 50 per cent, with depression in 28 per cent. However, half of female PRHOs show clinical depression. (Firth-Cozens, 1990). According to Johnson (1992), 79 per cent of PRHOs show emotional distress at some time during the year.

In the Tavistock project (Hale and Hudson, 1992) twenty SHOs were studied in depth. Five showed no evidence of stress, in five the findings were equivocal, but ten showed clear signs of maladaptive behaviour. Those from medical families appeared to cope better and those most distressed were five overseas doctors in their thirties or forties – in contrast to the British graduates who were in their early twenties. One of the most frequently acknowledged causes of stress was poor relations with seniors.

Although stress in other grades of staff is less well documented, above-average levels can be demonstrated at all grades, with women having higher rates than men (Hsu and Marshall, 1987). Among GPs, women show more free-floating anxiety and depression than men. In women a major source of stress appears to be the conflict between personal life and work. This stress is maximal in the later stages of training and early in the consultant career. There is a poor perception of part-time training in many specialities and women following this path often feel under-valued. Status has little influence on career choice in women, who often opt for low status non-career grades. Married women doctors show less stress than the unmarried, in contrast to the general population. Single women doctors are more likely to be depressed than those who are married and five times more likely to be seriously depressed than male doctors (Hsu and Marshall, 1987). Bynoe (1994) in a recent Yorkshire study confirmed the higher rates in single as compared to married women, with over half of the single women showing significant psychological disturbance. Single women moved more frequently and had less strong social networks and consequently they found it hard to establish networks when they settled into senior posts.

Women may also be able to separate the worries about work and home more effectively than men. If each contains sufficient rewards to provide positive as well as negative effects then buffering of the anxiety may occur (Stewart and Salt, 1981). It seems that marriage provides emotional support. Emotion-focused support (sympathy), however, does not always work and problem-focused support is more effective in stress relief. This might explain why emotional distress rates in dual medical marriages are half those in non-dual marriages. Perhaps the non-medical spouse provides support that is not problem focused whereas the medical spouse can add an understanding of the technicalities which may facilitate resolution.

Women doctors die on average ten years earlier than their male counterparts, the opposite of what happens in the general population. One factor here is the suicide rate among female physicians, which is significantly higher than among male doctors and four times higher than that of the age-matched female population (Heim, 1991). Training grade doctors identify relations with seniors as highly stressful. The senior doctor is often judged as remote, critical, and judgemental. From undergraduate days teaching is often by terror, with criticism if not ridicule rather than praise or encouragement. Many juniors complain that they never know how they are doing or how they are regarded because they only hear when they have done something wrong. Do not think, however, that drug and alcohol abuse, suicide, depression, and stress disorders are confined to junior doctors; they are at least as common in senior staff. Caplan (1994) recently demonstrated alarming rates in consultants and established GPs. There may be less sympathy for senior NHS managers, who show comparable rates.

Alcohol abuse is a common behavioural response to stress, and male PRHOs show a pattern of increased drinking. Allibone, Oakes and Shannon (1981) found evidence of this particularly in GPs. Murray (1976), in a study of Scottish doctors, found that the rates of admission for alcohol dependence were two to seven times higher among doctors than among controls of comparable social status.

The evidence for differential suicide rates between different specialities is difficult to obtain but it does appear that anaesthetists, radiologists, pathologists, and psychiatrists have higher rates and paediatricians have lower rates. Major sources of stress are in the area of patient satisfaction and the closely related doctor satisfaction. Doctors come to rely on patient praise and gratitude to sustain them in their work. The first complaint by a patient can be devastating and if this is followed by formal enquiry and possibly suspension or disciplinary proceedings the effects can be seriously disabling. The increasing penchant for litigation almost totally ignores the effect upon the doctor. Some distinguished doctors, particularly obstetricians, have given up clinical practice following litigation over cases in which their colleagues believed them to be blameless.

Sutherland and Cooper (1992) have demonstrated declining levels of job satisfaction among GPs and a recent BMA survey found that two-thirds of doctors believed they were experiencing a decline in job satisfaction. Forty per cent of the 1981 cohort to medical school now regret choosing medicine as a career and one in five of British graduates is no longer practising in the UK within five years of graduation.

Marital breakdown is regrettably common in doctors and the hours, the work intensity, the closed nature of medical communities, and the immediacy of the demands are undoubtedly factors in this. Increasing numbers of students are married; their wives anticipate no problems in their future role and look forward to improved economic and social status. In North America the spouse often provides financial support throughout medical school – a state that may soon be more common in the UK. After graduation the wives report their husbands professionally competent and successful but distant, rigid, controlling, and uncomfortable in dealing with feelings in marital and family relationships. Strategies the doctor adopts to avoid open conflict include prescribing medication for the wife, ignoring her frustration, and spending more time at work. The influential journal *McCalls Magazine* published an article entitled 'Never marry a doctor', which said, 'physicians are poor husbands, poor fathers, absent companions, prima donnas and about as useless in bed as an electric blanket with the power off'.

SUICIDE

Doctors have a high rate of suicide compared to the general population. They do of course have access to the means of suicide and a good understanding of their likely success. The Office of Population Censuses and Surveys for the years 1973–1983 shows that doctors have a 72 per cent greater risk of suicide than the general population. Compared to others of the same social class the risk for doctors is even greater. The rates for overseas graduates in medicine is greater still. This high suicide mortality for medical practitioners is a worldwide phenomenon (British Medical Association, 1993). The problem appears to be greatest among women, younger practitioners, and certain medical specialities such as anaesthesia (Harrington, 1987), radiology (Matanoski *et al.*, 1975), pathology (Harrington and Shannon, 1975), and psychiatry (Rich and Pitts, 1980). The SMR for single medical women aged between 16 and 60 years is 182 for external injury or poisoning and 371 for suicide. The Metropolitan Life Insurance Company of New York reported in 1974 that of 652 deaths among anaesthetists 20 per cent were due to suicide.

Harrington and his colleagues (Hall, Harrington and Aw, 1991) showed that pathologists had an excess mortality from suicide compared to the general population. The SMR for suicide in pathologists was 265 compared with an SMR of 176 among other medical practitioners in 1955–1973. The excess was found in both sexes. Blachly, Disher and Roshiner (1968) reported that suicide was lowest in paediatricians, with 10/100,000, and highest among psychiatrists, who had a rate of 61/100,000; though the methodology of this study has been questioned, no one has disputed this polarity. Rich and Pitts (1980) provides evidence to support the high rate among psychiatrists.

MORBIDITY

Chambers (1992) in a recent study of the lifestyle of GPs compared them with teachers and found that fewer GPs were current smokers and fewer drank more than 21 units of alcohol per week. Fewer GPs than teachers took regular exercise (13 per cent cf. 20 per cent). More of the GPs had taken no sickness absence in the prior three years (57 per cent cf. 17 per cent) and fewer reported exhaustion after work (53 per cent cf. 71 per cent). Teachers were more likely to be overweight, had a higher score for anxiety and depression, and male teachers were more likely to report an excessive alcohol intake.

Cooper's survey (Cooper, Rout and Faragher, 1989) of GPs' mental health, job satisfaction, and job stress was based on a large sample and reported that female GPs had lower scores for free-floating anxiety, depression, and psychosomatic symptoms than a normative UK population. Male GPs had higher scores for free-floating anxiety and those with a large number of stressors were more likely to show lack of mental 'well-being'. A second survey three years later, after the introduction of the new contract of employment for GPs, suggested that they were experiencing more stress, less job satisfaction, and poorer mental health than at the time of the first survey.

Spurgeon and Harrington (1989), reviewing the literature on the health of junior doctors, concluded, 'It is difficult to escape the conclusion that certain aspects of the junior doctor's job appear to be contributing to a high incidence of mental health problems.' A recent study by Caplan (1994) showed high scores on the GHQ, indicative of emotional distress, in principals in general practice, consultants, and health service managers.

ALCOHOL AND DRUGS

Abuse of alcohol and drugs may be adopted by doctors as a means of dealing with the high levels of stress in their lives. Until shortly after the Second World War a small group of doctors and others associated with medicine, such as pharmacists, nurses, and dentists, were the occupational groups most commonly addicted to controlled drugs. The wider availability of 'street drugs' has had little effect upon the pattern of abuse within the profession, for doctors use mainly alcohol or prescription drugs.

Vaillant, Brighton and McArthur (1970) were able to follow a sample of college students for twenty years and found that those who became doctors were more likely than other professionals to have poor marriages, to abuse alcohol, and to use sleeping pills, amphetamines, or tranquillizers. There is little doubt that medical students drink excessively but it is not clear that in this they differ from students in other faculties. Male medical students reported a mean alcohol consumption of about 20 units per week and females between 11.4 and 13.6 units per week. Nearly one-quarter of students exceeded 'safe' limits (defined as 35 units per week for men and 21 units per week for women) and more than half recognized that their academic performance had at times been impaired by alcohol. Firth (1986) found that 20 per cent of students in her study group admitted drinking heavily and that 48 per cent of the students had increased their alcohol intake during the previous two years in medical school.

A significant number of doctors who have later difficulties, including referral to the conduct committee of the GMC, have a history of excessive drinking in medical school. There are studies in the USA and other countries which indicate a high level of alcohol use among doctors but there is no clear evidence that doctors drink more than some other stressed professional groups (Clare, 1990). One recent report suggests that the great excess of alcohol-related problems in Scottish male doctors is largely due to a cohort of doctors over 45 years of age. They suggest that the younger generation have heeded advice on safe drinking (Harrison and Chick, 1994) but this may prove to be an optimistic view. Doctors have access to drugs and their income enables them to support a high alcohol intake but there is still no clear evidence that as a result they greatly exceed the level of abuse of these substances found in other groups. The main difference is that doctors impaired by alcohol or other drugs may be incompetent and thus place their patients at risk.

MENTAL ILLNESS

Doctors may well be at less risk of many mental disorders than the general population, for they have been selected by their academic ability and their commitment has been tested over a period of years. Studies of morbidity show that early in their career some doctors come to attention because of stress-related symptoms, anxiety, and depression of a situational type. Later they come into conflict with their employers or with the General Medical Council because of drug or alcohol abuse, major depressive illness, or severe anxiety-related disorders.

Frank schizophrenia is probably less common than in the general population. Although acute schizophrenia-like episodes are often recoverable and a return to practice may be possible, chronic schizophrenia is almost always incompatible with medical practice.

Recurrent manic depressive illness may prove difficult to manage but where a doctor is compliant with treatment continued practice should not carry a risk to patients. The dementing disorders usually require an early removal from practice. It is of course essential to identify treatable and potentially reversible disorders. Among the most tragic situations are doctors who have experienced severe head injury. The risk of accident is significantly higher for doctors than for the general population. In some, alcohol or drugs may play a part but high mileage and exhaustion are more common factors. A junior doctor after a long and busy shift may wish to drive home, or often to previous hospital where their friends are, and is at risk of falling asleep at the wheel. The same may apply to an overworked doctor, whose stressed state may result in such impairment of concentration that an accident occurs. The facilities for the treatment of acute head injuries have vastly improved and the prospects of survival for those reaching hospital are good. Unfortunately rehabilitation facilities have not shown a commensurate improvement and residual memory or learning difficulties are common. There are few posts in medicine where a graduated return to work without supervision is possible and cognitive neuropsychological rehabilitation is rarely available. Many patients after head injury have not only memory and learning problems but a significant degree of disinhibition and impaired impulse control which may render them unsuitable for clinical work. Given individually designed rehabilitation programmes, return to clinical work may be possible even after severe injury with residual neurological damage.

We now accept that those directly involved in the care or 'rescue' of individuals from major disasters may suffer from post-traumatic stress disorder (PTSD). Ambulance men and firemen are now recognized as at risk but there is less readiness to recognise that nurses and doctors exposed to horrific sights and expected to maintain professional detachment may develop symptoms of anxiety and frank PTSD.

A general practitioner was called to the house of a man who was known to be depressed and was threatening his wife and children. She arrived to find that the man was holding a shotgun to the head of one of the children and his wife was in such a state of distress that she collapsed and was assisted to the bedroom by the doctor. Meanwhile the police had arrived as a result of a call from a neighbour and a state of siege was established. There were shots from the house and the doctor was convinced that the man had killed one of the children and that she might be herself killed. The man came upstairs and after more than an hour of rambling conversation turned the gun on himself splashing blood and brain substance over the doctor.

She assisted in dealing with the aftermath but was too aroused to sleep that night and the following night had disturbed sleep.

Seventy-two hours after the event she became extremely agitated, had flashbacks of the suicide and felt afraid to leave her house. At night she suffered nightmares in which she herself was about to be killed. The full picture of post traumatic stress disorder developed but her colleagues were only marginally sympathetic urging that as an experienced doctor she should be able to cope with such events. She managed to continue in practice but began to use alcohol to enable her to complete her rounds and used heavy doses of sedatives to achieve sleep. Three months after the incident she was involved in a road traffic accident and was seriously injured and had to spend three months in hospital. It was during this time that her PTSD came to light and treatment was instituted.

DOCTORS AS PATIENTS

Reference has already been made to the reluctance shown by doctors to accept the patient role. There is often delay in seeking help. In Allibone's survey (Allibone, Oakes and Shannon, 1981) 46.4 per cent of a random sample admitted delay in seeking help for illness in the previous three years and more than one-quarter of hospital doctors and over a third of GPs self-treated illness. When the illness is emotional or drug related the reluctance is even more marked. Vincent (1969) claimed that 'all [studies] concur in the extreme reluctance of physicians to admit and to seek help for emotional problems'. A study of doctors with drink problems reported a delay in seeking treatment of over six years (Brooke, Edwards and Taylor, 1991). When they do seek help they frequently seek a consultation outside the normal channels, they may wish to participate in the consultation, discussing possible diagnosis and treatment, and as 'special patients' may expect special treatment, such as out-patient treatment where hospitalization would normally be required or expect to be able to come and go perhaps while continuing their practice. Their compliance with treatment is notoriously poor and they frequently prematurely discharge themselves from care. They are reluctant to attend clinics or to stay in hospital wards where they are known to staff and possibly to other patients. This reluctance is especially marked where the ward or unit specializes in the treatment of mental disorder.

Any patient is vulnerable and virtually stripped of their identity when in a hospital wheelchair or garbed in a dressing gown. A senior member of the staff of the hospital often finds it very difficult to cope with the jocularity and familiarity of many staff, which might be barely acceptable between total strangers. The senior professor of a medical school was admitted in some discomfort into the teaching hospital where he worked and was greeted by a probationer nurse who announced, 'I am Maisie. Do you want me to call you Charles or Charlie?'

The major preoccupations of most doctors entering care are their anxieties about confidentiality and privacy. Despite the central place of confidentiality in medical ethics, medical networks can become leaky sieves. There is a tendency to discuss patients, including colleagues, on the erroneous assumption that medical confidences may be shared with professional colleagues since they will respect the confidence. Such discussions may take place in the presence of other 'trusted' team members and sometimes it is assumed that wives fall into this category or somehow do not absorb confidential information. Any patient has the right to confidentiality and the assurance that information will be shared only on a need-to-know basis within the clinical team. Information about a patient, including the fact that the individual is at a given time actually a patient, is strictly confidential and may be disclosed only with the full and informed consent of the patient and only to the extent that is necessary for the purpose. In the past the sickness absence of doctors was dealt with confidentially by the District or Regional Medical Officer; now a doctor on extended sick leave is likely to be contacted by a non-medical personnel officer who will suggest a 'chat' with the consultant caring for the sick doctor. Attempts to arrange hospital treatment for a sick doctor at a hospital in another location involve the negotiation of an extra contractual referral (ECR), which may mean dealing with several non-medical employees of the trust members. Although there is a requirement of confidentiality there is a realistic fear that the matter will be discussed outside the bounds of 'need to know.'

The Chief Medical Officer's report *Maintaining Medical Excellence* (DoH, 1995) urges doctors to ensure that 'concern about colleagues is brought to the attention of the appropriate authority' and goes on to 'consider that the professional responsibility to monitor the standard of colleagues' professional performance needs to be reinforced to all doctors'. There appears to have been some misunderstanding of the GMC guidance which states, 'Furthermore, it is any doctor's duty, where the circumstances so warrant, to inform an appropriate person or authority ...' In other words doctors have a responsibility to ensure that steps are taken to protect the public if a colleague appears to be impaired but this may involve ensuring that the individual receives appropriate care rather than being reported to 'an appropriate authority'. How can appropriate care be arranged?

CURRENT ARRANGEMENTS FOR THE CARE OF SICK DOCTORS IN THE UNITED KINGDOM

All doctors should register with a GP whom they will be willing to consult in time of need. It is impossible to avoid some degree of self-diagnosis but self-prescription should be discouraged. This will require a considerable change of attitude but is unlikely to be achieved by punitive sanctions. The criminalization of self-prescription would simply drive it underground.

At the present time occupational health services are very patchy in the National Health Service and they are not seen as a treatment service. In future they may have some role in the early identification and prevention of mental ill health.

The treatment resources of the NHS should be available to any doctor but where there is a problem of impaired competence or drug or mental problems then treatment and any in-patient admission required may need to be arranged in a centre away from the usual place of employment. This raises the many problems associated with extra contractual referrals most of which could be avoided by an agreement, administered by Clinical Directors, to operate on a 'knock for knock' basis. Where the doctor is unable or unwilling to seek treatment and a risk to patients is possible then, in hospital, the 'three wise men' procedure (HC[82]13) may be invoked. There is a comparable procedure in general practice through the Local Medical Committee (*British Medical Journal*, 1986). The chairman of the professional panel or 'three wise men' is appointed locally and may be consulted in confidence by anyone concerned about a colleague. If the chairman agrees that a problem exists it may be possible to resolve this by the doctor concerned agreeing to take sick leave and seek appropriate treatment. If there is a risk and the doctor refuses to take appropriate action then a panel of three is convened and having decided on the appropriate action discuss this with the doctor before informing 'the appropriate authority'. Under this procedure no formal records are maintained and where the system is working well the majority of cases are resolved without risk to patients or resort to formal proceedings. Unfortunately the system has in the past been compromised by the confidentiality and secrecy that surround it and in many districts has never worked well. The future of this mechanism is now in doubt mainly because of the trust structure and the changed role of the Directors of Public Health, who as District Medical

Officers played a crucial role in supporting the chairman of the 'professional committee' as it was usually known.

There is reluctance to invoke the 'three wise men' procedure in those areas where it is not well established or is regarded with suspicion because of fears regarding confidentiality. It is in these cases that the National Counselling Service for Sick Doctors (NCSSD) is particularly useful. This organisation was set up in 1985 to provide an accessible, confidential, and non-coercive counselling service to doctors unable or unwilling to recognize their need to seek treatment. The initial contact may be made by the doctor, by a colleague, or by a close relative and is made by telephoning a central contact number that is listed each week on the salary page of the *British Medical Journal*. At this stage only the speciality and the area in which the doctor practises is required and the caller is provided with the name of an adviser from the same speciality but a different geographical area. The caller then contacts the adviser by telephone and the doctor concerned helps to arrange appropriate consultation and treatment. Advisers have access through the Royal College of Psychiatrists to a list of over 200 psychiatric counsellors who are willing to assist. If the initial contact is not made by the doctor concerned then the adviser has the delicate task of approaching the doctor and attempting to ascertain whether or not a problem exists. If at this stage the doctor rejects the offer of help then the adviser encourages the doctor to make further contact but if this is not taken up within a reasonable time the original informant is advised.

All of the doctors involved in the NCSSD give their services free. This service, which is available to all medical practitioners, now deals with over 400 referrals each year. The Association of Anaesthetists operate an independent scheme, which started before the NCSSD but operates on the same lines.

The Nuffield Provincial Hospitals Trust (1996) made an important series of recommendations for the improvement and better coordination of existing services. The report reviewed the evidence of stress-related morbidity in the profession and the needs of doctors, and concluded that in terms of the conservation of a scarce resource special services for doctors can be justified. It was recognised that it was important to reduce avoidable stress, if necessary by changing working conditions and the nature of the job, as well as providing adequate services for those who fall ill. The central proposal of the report was the creation of a network of independent regional bodies to be responsible for:

- reviewing the services available for doctors with health problems
- identifying steps that should be taken to improve working conditions where these are found to be unsatisfactory
- drawing up recommendations for a longer term programme of improvements
- monitoring progress
- providing information about existing services and developments, both local and national
- publishing an annual report.

These regional bodies should be fully independent of local health authorities and providers, in order to establish their impartiality *vis-à-vis* the interests of employers. These proposals apply to doctors and could be rapidly implemented and could serve as a model for other groups in the NHS.

THE GENERAL MEDICAL COUNCIL

The council is concerned with the registration of medical practitioners and the regulation of the profession, particularly with regard to the protection of the public. For many doctors it is seen as a semijudicial body which can deprive them of their livelihood and though widely respected is also widely feared. It deals with serious professional misconduct and recently its powers were extended to enable it to deal with doctors whose standards of performance consistently fall below those expected of the profession.

When a complaint is made against a doctor there is a preliminary screening of the evidence and if it appears to the medical screener that the problems may arise from ill health then the doctor can be required to be examined by two independent specialists, usually psychiatrists, who will report to the Health Committee, who may then order appropriate medical supervision and rehabilitation of the sick doctor. Where there is a reluctance on the part of the doctor to comply or the seriousness of the situation so demands, the doctor may be required to appear before the full Health Committee. So long as the complaint is being dealt with by the Health Committee the proceedings remain confidential.

ALCOHOL AND DRUG ADDICTION

Doctors with serious problems of addiction may benefit from membership of one of the British Doctors' and Dentists' Groups. There are a number of local groups which operate on a basis of strict confidentiality in a similar manner to Alcoholics Anonymous and aim at total abstention. They may be contacted through the Medical Council on Alcoholism (0171 487 4445).

An independent but related group have set up a National Intervention Scheme which will provide direct clinical service and supervision. Dr Ian M. Joiner can provide further information on this scheme (01252 316976).

The Royal College of General Practitioners and the British Medical Association are each independently experimenting with a number of telephone helplines which may eventually become available on a national basis. The rising concern about sick doctors is generating more separate schemes than can be mentioned here and the need is now for some coordination of these disparate efforts.

CONCLUSION

The National Health Service is the largest employer in the United Kingdom, there are not enough doctors or nurses available to meet currently identifiable needs, and yet there is little evidence that the employer is prepared to provide adequate care for the carers. Any commercial undertaking of comparable size would make a substantial investment to improve working conditions, to investigate causes of sickness, and to provide effective treatment and rehabilitation services. Highly trained health professionals are too scarce a resource and take too long to train for any employer to take risks of damaging them. It is high time the Department of Health took on the responsibility for providing proper care for the NHS work force.

REFERENCES

Allibone, A., Oakes, D. and Shannon, H.S. (1981) The health and health care of doctors. *Journal of the College of General Practitioners*, **31**, 728–34.

Anon (1974) Mortality of anaesthesiologists. *Statistical Bulletin, Metropolitan Life Insurance Company*, **55**, 5–8.

Ashley-Miller, M. and Lehmann, M. (1993) Alternative career paths for doctors. *British Medical Journal*, **307**, 886.

Balajaran, R. (1989) Inequalities in health within the health sector. *British Medical Journal*, **299**, 822–5.

Blachly, P.H., Disher, W. and Roshiner, G. (1968) *Bulletin of Suicidology*, December, 1–18.

British Medical Association (1992) *Stress and the Medical Profession*, BMA, London.

British Medical Association (1993) *The Morbidity and Mortality of the Medical Profession*, BMA, London.

British Medical Journal (1986) LMC scheme to help sick doctors. **293**, 899–900.

Brooke, D., Edwards, G. and Taylor, C. (1991) Addiction as an occupational hazard; 144 doctors with drug and alcohol problems. *British Journal of Addiction*, **86**, 1613–17.

Bynoe, G. (1994) Stress in women doctors. *British Journal of Hospital Medicine*, **51**, 267–8.

Caplan, R.P. (1994) Stress, anxiety and depression in hospital consultants, general practitioners and senior health managers. *British Medical Journal*, **309**, 1261–3.

Chambers, R. (1992) Health and lifestyle of general practitioners and teachers. *Occupational Medicine*, **42**, 69–78.

Clare, A.W. (1990) The alcohol problem in universities and the professions. *Alcohol and Alcoholism*, **25**, 277–85.

Collee, J. (1993) Brace against time. *The Observer*, Life Supplement, 26 December, p. 27.

Cooper, C.L., Rout, U. and Faragher, B. (1989) Mental health, job satisfaction and job stress among general practitioners. *British Medical Journal*, **298**, 366–70.

Department of Health & Social Security (1986) Prevention of harm to patients resulting from physical or mental disability of hospital or community medical or dental staff. DHSS HC(82)13, London.

DoH (1995) Maintaining Medical Excellence. Department of Health, London.

Firth, J. (1986) Levels and sources of stress in medical students. *British Medical Journal*, **292**, 1177–80.

Firth-Cozens, J. (1990) Sources of stress in women junior house officers. *British Medical Journal*, **301**, 89–91.

Freudenberger, H.J. (1984) Staff burn-out. *Journal of Social Issues*, **30**, 159–65.

Hale, R. and Hudson, L. (1992) The Tavistock study of young doctors: report of the pilot phase. *British Journal of Hospital Medicine*, **47**, 452–64.

Hall, A., Harrington, J.M. and Aw, T.C. (1991) Mortality study of British pathologists. *American Journal of Industrial Medicine*, **20**, 83–9.

Harrington, J.M. (1987) The health of anaesthetists. *Anaesthesia*, **42**, 131–2.

Harrington, J.M. and Shannon, H.S. (1975) Mortality of pathologists and medical laboratory technicians. *British Medical Journal*, **i**, 329–32.

Harrison, D. and Chick, J. (1994) Trends in alcoholism among male doctors in Scotland. *Addiction*, **89**, 1613–17.

Heim, E. (1991) Job stressors and coping in health professions. *Psychotherapy and Psychosomatics*, **55**, 90–9.

Hsu, K. and Marshall, V. (1987) Prevalence of depression and distress in a large sample of Canadian residents, interns and fellows. *American Journal of Psychiatry*, **144**, 1561–6.

Johnson, W.D.K. (1992) Stresses and stress outcomes in junior house officers. Unpublished doctoral thesis.

Matanoski, G.M., Seltser, R., Sartwell, P.E. *et al.* (1975) *American Journal of Epidemiology*, **101**, 199–210.

Menzies, I. (1960) Institutional defence against anxiety. *Human Relations*, **13**, 95–121.

Murray, R.M. (1976) Alcoholism amongst male doctors in Scotland. *Lancet*, **ii**, 729–31.

Nuffield Provincial Hospitals Trust (1996) Taking care of doctors' health. NPHT, London.

Office of Population Censuses and Surveys (1986) *Occupational mortality 1979–80, 1982–83*, HMSO, London.

Rich, C.L. and Pitts, F.N. (1980) Suicide by psychiatrists: a study of medical specialists among 18,730 consecutive physician deaths during a five year period, 1967–72. *Journal of Clinical Psychiatry*, **41**, 261–3.

Richings, J.C., Khara, G.S. and McDowell, M. (1986) Suicide in young doctors. *British Journal of Psychiatry*, **149**, 475–8.

Secombe, J., Ball, J. and Patch, A. (1993) The price of commitment; nurses' pay, careers and prospects. Report No. 251, Institute of Manpower Studies, London.

Spurgeon, A. and Harrington, J.M. (1989) Work performance and health of junior doctors – a review of the literature. *Work and Stress*, **3**, 117–28.

Stewart, A.J. and Salt, P. (1981) Life stress, life styles, depression and illness in adult women. *Journal of Personal and Social Psychology*, **40**, 1063–9.

Sutherland, V.J. and Cooper, C.L. (1992) Job stress, satisfaction and mental health among general practitioners before and after introduction of new contract. *British Medical Journal*, **304**, 1545–8.

Vaillant, G.E., Brighton, J.R. and McArthur, C. (1970) Physicians use of mood altering drugs. A 20-year follow-up report. *New England Journal of Medicine*, **282**, 365–70.

Vincent, M.O. (1969) Physicians and alcoholism. *Reports Alcohol*, **27**, 5.

6

Measuring stress, coping, and burnout in health care professionals

Jerome Carson and Sally Hardy

INTRODUCTION

The massive explosion in research activity in recent years into stress, coping, and burnout in health care professionals has been fuelled by two major factors. First, practitioners are naturally interested in issues that directly concern them. Thus the burnout field was largely driven in the early years by practitioners rather than researchers (Maslach and Schaufeli, 1993). Second, the accumulating series of empirical studies on professional groups has developed further momentum. Most research studies end with the conclusion that more research needs to be carried out on the topic, and researchers in this field have not been found wanting! Chapter 2 of this book highlights some of the background literature and developments within stress studies of health professionals.

The issue of how to measure stress, assess coping skills, and determine levels of burnout is a central one for research. In this chapter we review the measurement of stress, coping, and burnout. We focus particularly on the use of self-report measures as these constitute the main measurement tools employed. We then look at alternative methods, such as examining absenteeism and turnover at work. We look at assessment of work climate and job satisfaction. While self-report measures have their own methodological shortcomings, they are likely to remain a major research method for obtaining individual perceptions of stress and its effects. We conclude that researchers will need to be more discriminating in their selection of measures for studies. Not only will they have to select measures that are psychometrically robust, but they will also have to adopt designs that add to the scientific literature in a meaningful manner. There is a need for more theoretically driven research. We end by describing a tentative model that incorporates stress, coping, and burnout within a more comprehensive explanatory framework than most research has used to date.

SELF-REPORT QUESTIONNAIRES

The humble questionnaire is probably the single most common research tool in the social sciences according to Fife-Schaw (1995). Questionnaires have a number of advantages over other research methods. First, they are relatively low in researcher cost, unlike interviewer studies. Second, combinations of questionnaires can easily be assembled to answer most research questions. Third, the method itself is quite simple, and has a long research tradition (Oppenheim, 1992). Of course, questionnaires have their own problems such as response bias (Rust and Golombok, 1989). Guilbert (1992) lists the following problems: leniency errors, central tendency, halo effects, logical errors, contrast errors, proximity errors. In evaluating any questionnaire it is critical to be aware of its reliability, validity, and utility.

EVALUATING A QUESTIONNAIRE'S EFFECTIVENESS

Streiner (1993) has provided an invaluable checklist for evaluating questionnaires. He starts by stating that it is important to know where items have come from. He notes that 'borrowing from one source is plagiarism, but taking from two or more is research' (Streiner, 1993, p.141). Items should be checked for endorsement frequency, restrictions in range, comprehension, lack of ambiguity, and for possible offensive or value-laden content.

Reliability refers to the precision or accuracy of a questionnaire. It is assessed in three main ways: (i) internal consistency, (ii) test re-test, and (iii) inter-rater agreement (if applicable).

Validity refers to whether a questionnaire actually measures what it is supposed to measure.

Face validity relates to whether a measure seems to be the specific domain under investigation.

Content validity concerns the scale covering all the relevant dimensions of a particular construct.

Concurrent criterion validity (sometimes referred to in Britain as concurrent correlational validity) assesses how the measure compares against similar measures of the same phenomenon.

Predictive validity relates to whether a score on a measure enables us to predict future behaviour.

Construct validity is established when additional research begins to build up a body of confirmatory evidence of the meaningfulness of the construct under investigation.

The *utility* of any questionnaire measure is evaluated by considering the time taken to complete it, the amount of training necessary to administer it, and the complexity of scoring it and interpreting the results.

MEASURING STRESS

A fundamental problem in measuring stress is the basic disagreement as to what stress actually is. Beehr (1995) points out, 'there is currently no accepted model of stress being used in the field' (Beehr, 1995, p. 50). Mazure and Druss (1995) provide a helpful historical account of stress and its relationship to psychiatric illness. Our concern in this chapter is more specifically with work stress, rather than the link with formal psychiatric illness. Some of our own work (Brown *et al.*, 1995), has utilized a simplified model of stress based on the work of Professor Cooper and his colleagues (Cooper, Sloan and Williams, 1988). This model looks at four stages in the stress response cycle (Figure 6.1).

Measuring stressors could take place in terms of evaluating specific work stressors, or in terms of stress outcomes. It seems reasonable to assume that each mental health profession experiences some stress that is unique to that profession. In Britain social workers are intimately involved in the operation of the Mental Health Act (1983) and if they have 'approved social worker status', they may be involved in the compulsory admission of the mentally ill into hospital. Participating in such admissions can be very stressful. Similarly, nurses have the greatest amount of face to face contact with patients during all phases of their illness and this is likely to constitute a specific occupational stress.

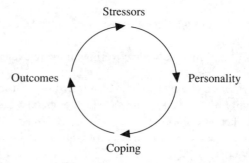

Figure 6.1 A simplified model of stress. Based on Cooper, Sloan and Williams (1988).

MEASURING SPECIfiC OCCUPATIONAL STRESSORS

How does one go about measuring specific occupational stressors? The generic approach would be to devise measures that could be used across several occupational groups. Cushway and her colleagues have developed the Mental Health Professionals Stress Scale (Nolan, Cushway and Tyler, 1995). This measure can be administered to any mental health profession, and their scores compared against scale norms. Most researchers have, however, adopted the specific approach. Hence Grey-Toft and Anderson (1981a,b), developed a measure of stress for nurses. Sweeney, Nichols and Kline developed a measure for occupational therapists (1991, 1993), whilst Deary and colleagues devised one specifically for doctors (Agius *et al.*, 1996).

Our own contribution to this field has been to develop specific measures of stress for mental health nurses. In Britain, there are two main areas of mental health nursing: ward or hospital-based nursing and community nursing (Nolan, 1993). In the days of asylum nursing, most nurses were based in hospitals but increasingly nurses are now working in the community (White, 1990). Initially we developed a measure of stress for community nurses called the CPN Stress Questionnaire (Carson, Bartlett and Croucher, 1991). More recently we have devised a measure for ward staff, the DCL stress scale (Carson *et al.*, 1996a).

The DCL stress scale comprises 30 items rated on a five-point distress scale. Factor analysis showed that five factors accounted for 65.8 per cent of the variance. These factors were: (i) patient demands, (ii) organizational and managerial issues, (iii) staffing, (iv) future concerns and (v) job satisfaction. In terms of Streiner's checklist (Streiner, 1993) this measure performs well. First, it underwent a rigorous process of item selection and item analysis. Second, it has high internal consistency and satisfactory test re-test reliability. Third, it has good face and content validity, plus reasonable concurrent criterion validity. Further work needs to be conducted to establish its predictive and construct validity. Fourth, it is quick to complete and easy to administer and score. Interpretation is helped by the availability of a detailed manual.

The work on ward-based nurses is important as it highlights the differing nature of stress on the ward compared to that in the community setting. In an earlier study (Fagin *et al.*, 1995) we demonstrated that it was more stressful to work in the community, but more satisfying. However, it is not just the level of stress that is different, as previously stated, it is the specific nature of the stressors. For hospital-based nurses the two greatest stressors were: inadequate staffing cover in potentially dangerous situations, and individual care being sacrificed due to lack of staff. In contrast the two top stressors identified by the community nurses were: not having facilities that clients can be referred on to, and knowing that there are likely to be long waiting lists for clients before they can get access to services (Carson *et al.*, 1995).

THE GENERAL HEALTH QUESTIONNAIRE

While it is clearly important to measure the level and nature of work stressors experienced by staff, it is also crucial to evaluate stress outcomes. One of the most widely used measures of psychological distress is the General Health Questionnaire (GHQ) (Goldberg and Williams, 1988). There are currently four versions of this scale with the title reflecting the number of items included. The largest study of NHS staff ever conducted used the GHQ-12. In our studies we have used the GHQ-28, as have some previous stress researchers (Cushway, 1992). Two scores are obtained from the GHQ – a total score and a caseness rating. Total scores for staff on the GHQ-28 tend to be in the range of 3 to 5, in contrast to the average scores of around 10 points for patients referred to psychologists in community settings (Carson and Brewerton, 1991). While the GHQ-28 breaks down into four subscales (anxiety and insomnia, somatic symptoms, social role functioning, and severe depression), scores on these subscales tend to be low in non-clinical samples, so the total score is preferred. Some researchers also use a different scoring method, the Likert method, which scores items on a 0–3 scale rather than the conventional 0–1 GHQ method.

The scale has been criticized for the use of the caseness criterion, which suggests that certain proportions of the population could be identified as psychiatric cases on the basis of their scoring (i.e. a score of 5 or more on the GHQ-28). In reality these people may be experiencing significant levels of psychological distress, yet very few will ever become psychiatric cases *per se*. Bowling (1995) describes the GHQ as the most commonly used international scale of general psychiatric morbidity across a wide range of patients. The reliability of the GHQ has been extensively investigated with test re-test correlations ranging from $r + 0.51$ to 0.90 (Goldberg and Williams, 1988). Internal consistency is also high, and the GHQ is impressive in its validity. The scale has good content validity, good concurrent criterion validity, and established construct validity (Berwick, Budman and Damico-White, 1987). The Crown Crisp Experiential Index was developed at the same time (Crown and Crisp, 1979). It is a similar screening measure, yet with few exceptions (Cooper, Rout and Faragher, 1989) the CCEI has been completely superseded in the work stress literature by the GHQ. In terms of its utility the GHQ is quick to administer and easy to score and interpret.

MEASURING COPING SKILLS

Pearlin and Schooler (1978) defined coping as any response to external life strains that serves to prevent, avoid or control emotional distress. This is similar to the definition provided by Lazarus and Folkman (1984), who argued that stress consists of three processes:

(1) Primary appraisal, the process of perceiving a threat.

(2) Secondary appraisal, the process of thinking of potential responses to that threat.

(3) Coping, the process of carrying out a response to a threat.

Coping is the process of responding to stress in such a way that the effects of the stressor are minimized. Pearlin and Schooler (1978) divided coping strategies into three main types:

(1) Responses that change the situation.

(2) Responses that change the meaning of the situation.

(3) Responses that control the stressful consequences after they have occurred.

An alternative perspective has been provided by Carver, Scheier and Weintraub (1989). Following Lazarus and Folkman they suggest there are three distinct types of coping: (i) problem-focused coping, (ii) emotion-focused coping, and (iii) disengagement coping. Just as there are several measures of stress, so there are several measures of coping. In this next section we will focus on only two. The first is the Cooper Coping Skills Scale, from the occupational stress indicator (Cooper, Sloan and Williams, 1988), and the second is the Coping Resources Inventory (Billings and Moos, 1981). These represent contrasting approaches to the assessment of coping skills.

The Cooper Coping Skills Scale comprises six separate subscales. These are: social support, which has four items, for example, 'seek support and advice from my superiors'; task strategies (seven items), such as 'reorganize my work'; logic (three items) – 'try to deal with the situation objectively in an unemotional way'; home and work relationships (four items) – 'having a home that is a refuge'; time (four items) – 'deal with problems immediately they occur'; involvement (six items) – 'look for ways to make the work more interesting'.

Scores are obtained for all six subscales with items rated on a frequency of occurrence basis: 1 = 'never used by me', to 6 = 'very extensively used by me'. Subscale scores can then be compared for sample groups. For instance comparing the scores of community and ward-based nurses from the Claybury CPN study (Fagin *et al.*, 1995) showed significant differences only in the use of task strategies and logic. Comparison of male and female staff revealed that women use significantly more social support than men, who in turn use logic significantly more than do women.The most popular coping strategies for all staff were having stable relationships, separating home from work, and recognizing their limitations. Other research workers who have used this scale have told Professor Cooper that rather than any of the six subscales, the most reliable measure is a total coping skills score (Cooper, 1996, personal communication). Indeed our research group found that if we divided our sample of 648 ward mental health nurses into high coping skills and low coping skills groups on the basis of a top and bottom percentile cut, the two groups showed significant differences in stress outcome measures. The high coping skills group had significantly lower stress levels on the GHQ-28 and on the Maslach emotional exhaustion subscale (Carson *et al.*, 1996b).

It would seem then that the more coping skills an individual uses, the lower will be their level of stress. Cooper, Sloan and Williams (1988) report data on the reliability and validity of the scale. Split half reliability of the scale ranges from $r = 0.07$ on logic to 0.59 on home and work relationships. Cooper partly attributes these low reliabilities to problems of the split half reliability calculation and also to the fact that the scale comes at the end of a very long battery of measures. Much more work needs to be conducted on the psychometric properties of this scale; our own research group will be reporting on this shortly. On a more positive note, the scale is easy to score and the manual has normative data for comparative purposes (Cooper, Sloan and Williams, 1988).

The Coping Resources Inventory (Moos, 1990) is the second measure under investigation. In this test the client is first asked to select the most stressful problem or situation that they have experienced in the last 12 months. A preliminary section with 10 items is then answered and is concerned with how the stress was appraised (e.g. 'Have you ever faced a problem like this before?'). Following this the main scale with 48 items is administered. The client is asked to think again about the initial problem identified and to indicate which strategies they use to deal with the situation. Strategies are rated on a four-point scale from no to yes, fairly often. The scale has eight subscales: logical analysis ('think of different ways to deal with the problem'); positive appraisal ('tell yourself things to make yourself feel better'); seeking support ('talk to your partner or relative about the problem); problem solving ('make a plan of action and follow it'); cognitive avoidance ('try to forget the whole thing'); acceptance ('feel that time would make a difference – the only thing to do is wait'); alternative rewards ('get involved in new activities'); emotional discharge ('take it out on other people when you feel angry or depressed'). Each subscale has six items. The scale takes about 15 minutes to complete and can be given as a self-report questionnaire or used as a structured interview. There are good normative data available and the scale has satisfactory internal consistency and test re-test reliability. While one might speculate that coping responses will vary depending on the nature of the major stressor identified, Moos (1990) reports that the scale shows high consistency over time, despite variations in stressors.

MEASURING BURNOUT

Unlike the concept of stress, burnout is a relatively recent addition to the research literature. The term itself was first described by Freudenberger (1974, 1975). Yet in the first major review of the concept, Perlman and Hartman (1982) claimed that there were more than 48 different definitions of burnout. The most widely accepted definition is that of Maslach and Jackson (1986): 'Burnout is a syndrome of emotional exhaustion, depersonalisation and reduced personal accomplishment that can occur among individuals who do people work of some kind' (Maslach and Schaufeli, 1993, p. 14). While Freudenberger concentrated more on the clinical description of the phenomenon of burnout, Maslach and her colleagues have adopted a more empirical approach (Farber, 1983). Farber points out that stress and burnout are not the same. Burnout he argues is not a result of stress *per se*, but of unmediated stress – a sense of being stressed with no escape. He further argues that the concepts differ in that stress can actually be a positive experience. However, Freudenberger (1983) claims that burnout can also have positive features, in that it may persuade the individual to do something about their situation. Maslach and Schaufeli (1993) point out that the level of burnout seems fairly stable over time. Its nature is more chronic than acute. Burnout leads to physical symptoms, to absenteeism and job turnover, whereas role conflict and lack of social support from colleagues are antecedents.

Burnout has almost exclusively been measured by self-report questionnaire assessment. The two major measures are Maslach's Burnout Inventory and Pines and Aronson's Burnout Measure.

The Maslach Burnout Inventory (MBI) (Maslach and Jackson, 1986) comprises 22 items that are rated on a seven-point frequency of occurrence basis. The scale has three separate and independent subscales. These are emotional exhaustion (9 items), e.g. 'I feel emotionally drained from my work'; depersonalization (5 items), 'I worry that this job is hardening me'; personal accomplishment (8 items), 'I feel I'm influencing other people's lives through my work'.

The internal consistency of the MBI is high ($r + 0.71$ to 0.90) with a normative sample of some 11,000 subjects. Test re-test reliability ranges from $r = 0.60$ to 0.80 for periods of up to one month. Emotional exhaustion is the most stable burnout dimension, whereas depersonalization is the least stable. Schaufeli, Enzman and Girault (1993) conclude that, while the MBI has good factorial and convergent validity, the concept of burnout overlaps so closely with depression and to a lesser degree with job satisfaction as to suggest it may not be an independent construct. Our previous research (Fagin *et al.*, 1995) found that community mental health nurses had significantly greater levels of personal accomplishment and experience significantly less depersonalization than their ward-based counterparts.

The MBI is scored in two ways. First, subscale scores are obtained. Second, each score is categorized as falling into a high, moderate or low group, based on

Table 6.1 High versus low emotional exhaustion

Mean scores	Maslach high emotional exhaustion (n = 359)	Maslach low emotional exhaustion (n = 307)	Significance level Mann–Whitney
Days absence	8.11	7.11	$p < 0.01$
General Health Questionnaire score (GHQ-28)	6.67	1.43	$p < 0.001$
Maslach depersonalization	9.92	3.32	$p < 0.001$
Maslach personal accomplishment	33.17	32.56	Not significant
Minnesota extrinsic job satisfaction	14.82	18.31	$p < 0.001$
Minnesota intrinsic job satisfaction	39.14	43.99	$p < 0.001$
Minnesota total job satisfaction	59.57	68.65	$p < 0.001$

cut-offs defined in the manual (Maslach and Jackson, 1986). Partial evidence for the validity of the subscale of emotional exhaustion is provided in Table 6.1. From a combined sample of 900 mental health nurses, 359 were found to score in the high burnout category, with 307 in the low range. Table 6.1 shows how both groups differ on a range of measures. The measures are: self-reported absence in the last 12 months; score on GHQ-28; Maslach depersonalization and personal accomplishment; the Minnesota Job Satisfaction Scale (Koelbel, Fuller and Misener, 1991).

The Burnout Measure (BM), is the second most widely employed questionnaire to measure burnout (Pines and Aronson, 1988). It comprises 21 items that are scored on a seven-point scale from never to always. A single burnout score is obtained. The internal consistency of the scale is high, ranging from $r + 0.91$ to 0.93. Test re-test reliability ranges from $r = 0.66$ to 0.89. Pines and Aronson presented data showing that intention to leave the job was significantly correlated with the BM score in social workers. They also demonstrated that turnover rates for staff in residential facilities for people with learning disabilities were higher in homes with elevated BM scores. Factor analytic studies reveal that there is only one dimension on the BM. This would appear to be the individual's level of exhaustion, which is also assessed on the MBI. Given that the MBI also assesses depersonalization and personal accomplishment, it would appear to be the preferred measure of burnout. This is also reflected in its much wider utilization in the research literature. Despite this, in a recent review of burnout in nursing, Duquette *et al.* (1994) recommended that a third measure of burnout – the Staff Burnout Scale for Health Professionals (Jones 1980, 1982) – be adopted as the most appropriate scale. Yet the psychometric properties of the SBS-HP have been criticized by Schaufeli, Enzman and Girault (1993). In our opinion the Maslach Burnout Inventory is the gold standard measure in this field. The third revision of the inventory has just been published and will no doubt lead to further research on the MBI (Maslach, Jackson and Leiter, 1996).

COMPOSITE MEASURES

An alternative approach to measuring work stress is to adopt one of the composite measures. Two of these measures will be described here. The advantages of such measures are that they are self-contained, and that researchers can use them on their own without the need for additional scales.

The Occupational Stress Indicator (Cooper, Sloan and Williams, 1988), has been developed in Britain. This self-report questionnaire measure is based on an expanded version of the model outlined earlier in this chapter (see Figure 6.1). The OSI has seven main questionnaires, with the whole batch taking between 45 minutes to one hour to complete. The questionnaire falls into four main sections.

Sources of stress

This is a 61 item questionnaire with six subscales covering stress factors intrinsic to the job, expectations, work relationships, career prospects, organizational structure, and the home–work interface.

Individual characteristics

This covers biographic and demographic items as well as two additional questionnaires. 'The way you behave generally' has 14 items covering attitude to living, style of behaviour, ambition, and a broad view of type A personality traits. The second, 'How you interpret events around you', has 12 statements which measure different aspects of control.

Coping with stress

This 28 item subscale was described earlier in the chapter and shows which six types of coping skills the individual uses most frequently.

The effects of stress on the individual and organization

Two questionnaires assess an individual's physical (12 items) and mental (18 items) health. Job satisfaction is assessed on a 22 item scale that covers satisfaction with achievement, with the job itself, with the organization, with organizational processes, and with work relationships. As this is a generic scale it can be used across the board in a variety of organizations. Increasing use in such settings will hopefully lead to the design of a more comprehensive manual with more data from different work settings. In Britain the OSI has already led to the publication of the first ever stress league table for health professionals (Rees and Smith, 1991). Interestingly at around the time that Professor Cooper was developing the OSI in Britain, Osipow and Spokane (1987) were developing the Occupational Stress Inventory in America. This scale covers three main dimensions of work stress. The first is occupational roles. This includes areas such as role ambiguity, role overload, and role boundaries. The second domain is personal strain, vocational strain, and interpersonal strain. Coping resources is the third area. This has four scales covering self-care, recreation, social support, and rational/cognitive coping. Data have been published on the validity of the scale (Osipow and Davis, 1988). This Inventory comprises 140 items and also has normative data on stress levels in several organizations.

Surprisingly, a lot of the research into stress and coping in health care professions has not utilized the two generic measures described above. The work of Rees and Smith (1991) is one of the few exceptions.

MEASURING ORGANIZATIONAL VARIABLES

While the composite measures described above looked at how individuals perceive their work environments, researchers have also focused on additional aspects
of the work environment. We will briefly mention three here: absenteeism and
turnover, work climate, and job satisfaction.

Absenteeism and turnover

It is often stated that absenteeism rates in organizations are an indicator of occupational stress and burnout. It has to be borne in mind, however, that not all
instances of sickness absence are stress related. Turnover within organizations is
again said to be an indicator of the stressfulness of the job. From a managerial
point of view, high turnover means additional costs in terms of recruiting, selecting, and training new staff. There is a need for researchers to utilize measures of
absence and turnover alongside more traditional psychometric measures of stress,
coping, and burnout.

Work climate

The atmosphere or therapeutic milieu of a health service setting is an important
factor in determining how staff feel about their workplace. It is, however, difficult
to assess work climate, as different groups of staff may have different needs. For
instance, in our research into stress in community nurses, one of the most stressful aspects of the job was having too many interruptions while trying to work in
the office (Carson *et al.*, 1994). These nurses did not feel that management valued
their needs and that they were often denied basic needs such as access to secretarial support or a good office base, which would have improved their perception of
the work climate. The Work Environment Scale (Moos, Insel and Humphrey,
1974) and the stress diagnostic survey (Ivancevich and Matteson, 1980) are both
methods of assessing work environments.

Job satisfaction

Low job satisfaction has been identified as a symptom of occupational stress.
Numerous studies have examined job satisfaction in different occupational groups. In
our own research we have utilized the Minnesota Job Satisfaction Scale to examine
job satisfaction levels in mental health nurses (Waite *et al.*, 1995). We found that
community mental health nurses had significantly higher levels of intrinsic and
total job satisfaction than ward-based colleagues. Both groups of nurses rated the
chance to do things for other people as the most satisfying aspect of their job. For
community nurses the chance to work alone was the next most satisfying aspect
of their job. Both groups of staff were dissatisfied with their working conditions
(especially community nurses) and with the way their employers treated them.

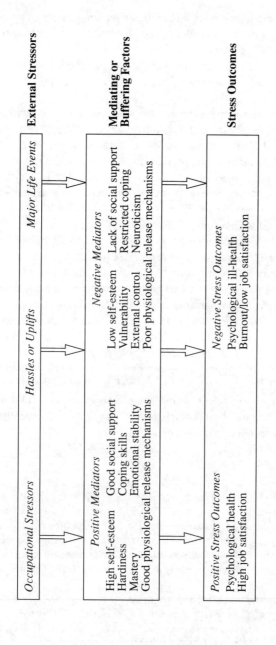

Figure 6.2 A model of the stress process.

CONCLUSIONS

In this chapter we have reviewed the measurement of stress, coping and burnout in health care professionals. We also described the initial model of stress that guided our earlier research endeavours. Our experience in investigating stress suggests that there is a clear need for a broader model of stress, which takes into account the complexity of the process. We outline just such a model below.

The model suggests that external stressors working on individuals come from three main sources (Figure 6.2). First, there are specific occupational stressors that can be measured by the various work stress scales. Second, there are a variety of minor or microstressors, sometimes referred as 'hassles' and 'uplifts' (Kanner *et al.*, 1981), which cumulatively can increase our stress levels. Third, we experience stress following major life events such as divorce or bereavements (Holmes and Rahe, 1967). The combined effects of these stressors will only lead to negative stress outcomes if we have insufficient resources to manage them. The critical factor in our model is what mediating or buffering factors an individual can call upon to minimize the effects of stress. We suggest that there are a number of possible mediating factors. We propose that high self-esteem, a good social support network, emotional stability, a sense of mastery and personal control, hardiness, good physiological release mechanisms, and a range of coping strategies will buffer the effects of stress. We believe that individuals who have such personal resources will experience better stress outcomes than individuals who lack them. We now need to test out our model through additional research.

We know that, as a group, health professionals are at risk of high levels of stress and burnout. The challenge now is to try and discover which mediating or buffering mechanisms best protect against the effects of stress and burnout. If we can establish which factors best protect staff we can deliver interventions to help and ultimately deliver better patient care.

REFERENCES

Agius, R., Blenkin, H., Deary, I. *et al.* (1996) Survey of perceived stress and work demands of consultant doctors. *Occupational and Environmental Medicine*, **53**, 217–24.

Beehr, T. (1995) *Psychological Stress in the Workplace*, Routledge, London.

Berwick, D., Budman, S. and Damico-White, J. (1987) Assessment of psychological morbidity in primary care: explorations with the General Health Questionnaire. *Journal of Chronic Disease*, **40**, 71–9.

Billings, A. and Moos, R. (1981) The role of coping responses and social resources in attenuating the stress of life events. *Journal of Behavioural Medicine*, **4**, 139–57.

Bowling, A. (1995) *Measuring Disease*, Open University Press, Buckingham.

Brown, D., Leary, J., Carson, J. *et al.* (1995) Stress in the community mental health nurse: The development of a measure. *Journal of Psychiatric and Mental Health Nursing*, **2** (1), 9–12.

Carson, J. and Brewerton, T. (1991) Out of the clinic into the classroom. *Adults Learning*, **2** (9), 256–7.

Carson, J., Bartlett, H. and Croucher, P. (1991) Stress and the community psychiatric nurse: A preliminary investigation. *Community Psychiatric Nursing Journal*, **11** (2), 8–12.

Carson, J., Bartlett, H., Brown, D. and Hopkinson, P. (1994) Findings from the qualitative study for community mental health nurses, in *Stress and Coping in Mental Health Nursing* (eds J. Carson, L. Fagin and S. Ritter), Chapman and Hall, London.

Carson, J., Leary, J., deVilliers, N. *et al.* (1995) Stress in mental health nurses: comparison of ward and community staff. *British Journal of Nursing*, **4** (10), 579–82.

Carson, J., deVilliers, N., O'Malley, P. *et al.* (1996a) Assessing stress in mental health nurses: reliability and validity of a new questionnaire. Submitted.

Carson, J., Cooper, C., Fagin, L. *et al.* (1996b) Coping skills in mental health nursing: do they make a difference? *Journal of Psychiatric and Mental Health Nursing*, **3** (3), 201–2.

Carver, C., Scheier, M. and Weintraub, J. (1989) Assessing coping strategies: a theoretically based approach. *Journal of Personality and Social Psychology*, **56** (2), 267–83.

Cooper, C., Sloan, J. and Williams, S. (1988) *Occupational Stress Indicator Management Guide*, NFER–Nelson, Windsor.

Cooper, C., Rout, U. and Faragher, B. (1989) Mental health, job satisfaction and job stress among general practitioners. *British Medical Journal*, **298**, 366–70.

Crown, S. and Crisp, A. (1979) *Manual of the Crown Crisp Experiential Index*. Hodder and Stoughton, London.

Cushway, D. (1992) Stress in clinical psychology trainees. *British Journal of Clinical Psychology*, **31**, 169–79.

Duquette, A., Kerouac, S., Sandhu, B. and Baudet, L. (1994) Factors related to nursing burnout: a review of empirical knowledge. *Issues in Mental Health Nursing*, **15**, 337–58.

Fagin, L., Brown, D., Bartlett, H. *et al.* (1995) The Claybury CPN stress study: is it more stressful to work in hospital or the community? *Journal of Advanced Nursing*, **22**, 1–12.

Farber, B. (ed.) (1983) *Stress and Burnout in the Human Service Professions*. Pergamon, New York.

Fife-Schaw, C. (1995) Questionnaire design, in *Research Methods in Psychology* (eds G. Breakwell, S. Hammond and C. Fife-Schaw), Sage Publications, London.

Freudenberger, H. (1974) Staff burnout. *Journal of Social Issues*, **30**, 159–65.

Freudenberger, H. (1975) The staff burnout syndrome in alternative institutions. *Psychotherapy: Theory, Research and Practice*, **12**, 72–83.

Freudenberger, H. (1983) Burnout: contemporary issues, trends and concerns, in *Stress and Burnout in the Human Service Professions* (ed. B. Farber), Pergamon, New York.

Goldberg, D. and Williams, P. (1988) *A User's Guide to the General Health Questionnaire*, NFER–Nelson, Windsor.

Grey-Toft, P. and Anderson, J. (1981a) The Nursing Stress Scale: development of an instrument. *Journal of Behavioural Assessment*, **3**, 11–23.

Grey-Toft, P. and Anderson, J. (1981b) Stress amongst hospital nursing staff: its causes and effects. *Social Science and Medicine*, **15**, 639–47.

Guilbert, J. (1992) *Educational Handbook for Health Personnel*. World Health Organisation, Geneva.

Holmes, T. and Rahe, R. (1967) The Social Readjustment Rating Scale. *Journal of Psychosomatic Research*, **11**, 213–18.

Ivancevich, J. and Matteson, M. (1980) *Stress and Work: a Managerial Perspective*, Scott Foresman, Park Ridge, IL.

Jones, J. (1980) *Preliminary Manual: The Staff Burnout Scale for Health Professionals*, London House Press, Park Ridge, IL.

Jones, J. (1982) *The Burnout Syndrome*. London House, New York.

Kanner, A., Coyne, J., Schaefer, C. and Lazarus, R. (1981) Comparison of two modes of stress management: daily hassles and uplifts versus major life events. *Journal of Behavioural Medicine*, **4**, 1–39.

Koelbel, P., Fuller, F. and Misener, T. (1991) Job satisfaction of nurse practitioners: an analysis using Herzberg's theory. *Nurse Practitioner*, **16** (4), 43–6.

Lazarus, R. and Folkman, S. (1984) *Stress, Appraisal and Coping*, Springer, New York.

Maslach, C. and Jackson, S. (1986) *The Maslach Burnout Inventory*, Consulting Psychologists Press, Palo Alto.

Maslach, C. and Schaufeli, W. (1993) Historical and conceptual development of burnout, in *Professional Burnout: Recent Developments in Theory and Research* (eds W. Schaufeli, C. Maslach and T. Marek), Taylor and Francis, Washington.

Maslach, C., Jackson, S. and Leiter, M. (1996) *The Maslach Burnout Inventory Manual*, 3rd edn, Consulting Psychologists Press, Palo Alto.

Mazure, C. and Druss, B. (1995) A historical perspective on stress and psychiatric illness, in *Does Stress Cause Psychiatric Illness* (ed. C. Mazure), American Psychiatric Association Press, Washington.

Moos, R. (1990) *Coping Responses Inventory Manual*, Psychological Assessment Resources, Odessa, FL.

Moos, R., Insel, P. and Humphrey, B. (1974) *Work Environment Scale*, Consulting Psychologists Press, Palo Alto.

Nolan, P. (1993) *A History of Mental Health Nursing*, Chapman and Hall, London.

Nolan, P., Cushway, D. and Tyler, P. (1995) A measurement scale for assessing stress among mental health nurses. *Nursing Standard*, **9**, 136–9.

Oppenheim, A. (1992) *Questionnaire Design, Interviewing and Attitude Measurement*. Pinter, London.

Osipow, S. and Davis, A. (1988) The relationship of coping resources to occupational stress and strain. *Journal of Vocational Behaviour*, **32**, 1–15.

Osipow, S. and Spokane, A. (1987) *Manual of the Occupational Stress Inventory*, Psychological Assessment Resources, Odessa, FL.

Pearlin, L. and Schooler, C. (1978) The structure of coping. *Journal of Health and Social Behaviour*, **19**, 2–21.

Perlman, B. and Hartman, A. (1982) Burnout: summary and future research. *Human Relations*, **35**, 283–305.

Pines, A. and Aronson, E. (1988) *Career Burnout: Causes and Cures*, Free Press, New York.

Rees, D. and Smith, S. (1991) Work stress in occupational therapists assessed by the Occupational Stress Indicator. *British Journal of Occupational Therapy*, **54** (8), 289–94.

Rust, J. and Golombok, S. (1989) *Modern Psychometrics: The Science of Psychological Assessment*, Routledge, London.

Schaufeli, W., Enzman, D. and Girault, N. (1993) Measurement of burnout: a review, in *Professional Burnout: Recent Developments in Theory and Research* (eds W. Schaufeli, C. Maslach and T. Marek), Taylor and Francis, Washington.

Streiner, D. (1993) A checklist for evaluating the usefulness of rating scales. *Canadian Journal of Psychiatry*, **38** (2), 140–8.

Sweeney, G., Nichols, K. and Kline, P. (1991) Factors contributing to work related stress in occupational therapists: results from a pilot study. *British Journal of Occupational Therapy*, **54** (8), 284–8.

Sweeney, G., Nichols, K. and Kline, P. (1993) Job stress in occupational therapists: an examination of causative factors. *British Journal of Occupational Therapy*, **56** (4), 140–5.

Waite, A., Oliver, N., Carson, J. and Fagin, L. (1995) Job satisfaction in mental health nursing: is community or ward based work more satisfying? *Psychiatric Care*, **2** (5), 167–70.

White, E. (1990) *The Third Quinquennial National Community Psychiatric Nursing Survey.* Department of Nursing, University of Manchester, Manchester.

PART TWO

The context of caring: facilitating workplace competence

7

David Sines

Much has been written about the subject of stress management in the workplace. Analysis of key concepts and variables that intervene in our daily work experiences may provide insight into the many causes of stress that health care professionals experience during the course of their everyday lives.

There is a considerable body of evidence to suggest that workplace cultures support (or fail to support) the competence of their workers. Staff are expected to strive for maximum productivity and efficiency (concepts that do not always accord with the 'caring philosophy' of the health service) and to promote health gain for their clients.

This chapter explores some of the key issues to be addressed in the quest for introducing a supportive workplace culture for employees. The process of preparing for change in the health service will also be considered as a constituent part of the organizational management task; levers for change will be described and extringent factors mapped. A central theme to the chapter will be the description of an organizational model that relies on the promotion of the 'competent workplace' that seeks to encourage front line staff to assume more control over their personal coping strategies.

Consequently the chapter aims to identify a framework designed to promote positive organizational practice within the context of a changing cultural environment. The chapter commences with an overview of service change and describes the context within which service change and patterns of staff adjustment may be considered.

THE PHILOSOPHY AND PRACTICE OF SERVICE PROVISION

In 1990 the Government published The National Health Service and Community Care Act, which provided the strategic framework for the provision of health and social care services in the UK. The Act unites the principles through which care is delivered between Health and Social Service agencies and encourages statutory agencies to form positive partnerships with consumers, their representatives, and with the voluntary and independent sectors to provide a positive choice in the provision of services. Emphasis was placed on the importance of developing partnerships between consumers, their representatives, and statutory agencies with the aim of promoting an open economy in care provision. As a result a new philosophy of care has emerged based on the principle that care should be shared with consumers and that, wherever possible, care should be provided as close to the patient's home as possible.

The enactment of this policy has now reduced patient/client dependency on in-patient or long-stay residential care in favour of seeking the development of a range of options based on local need which will be flexible enough to meet the demands of service provision required by local people in their neighbourhoods. The National Health Service (NHS) requires all health service providers to secure significant improvements in the way in which services are delivered to the population, emphasizing the promotion of positive health and the promotion of high quality care in the community. In order to provide these services, commissioners of health services must demonstrate that they provide a range of services to their clients and families as equal participants whenever decisions that will affect their lives are involved. Such principles now underpin the NHS philosophy and form the basis of the Government's Patient's Charter (Department of Health, 1992).

One other major issue for health service practitioners is the Government's issue of a mandate for the creation of NHS Trusts and GP Fundholding practices. In the 1990 Act NHS Trusts and Fundholding practices were encouraged to apply for independence within a centrally monitored National Health Service. The primary responsibility of these emergent agencies is to provide effective health care to a locally defined population and to ensure that they do so in accordance with user wishes. This role and function require that each NHS Trust and Fundholding practice gathers intelligence data to advise on the actual health care needs of the local population.

The emergence of Trusts and GP Fundholding practices has placed new demands on managers and their employees and now provides for the development of a management agenda characterized by local pay bargaining and autonomy in determining skill mix and qualification within the work force. The loosening up of central bureaucracy in the health service has presented some employees with additional conflicts as they strive to re-establish some degree of control over their pay and conditions of service and tenure within the work force.

Other influences that have been brought to bear on the health care agenda are:

- The growth of consumerism and non-statutory sector care in the mixed economy of service provision suggests a demand for more equal relationships between clients/patients and health care professionals. There is also a growing expectation that individuals will assume responsibility for their own health and lifestyles.
- Changes in social policy have placed increasing continuing care responsibilities on informal carers in the home. Demographic changes and economic demands are changing the nature of the family's caring role, which may be influenced by the number of women entering the labour market. Similarly the projected increase in the number of elderly persons requiring community care has also demanded additional nursing resources.
- Rapid technological and pharmacological developments, new patterns of disease and disability, and the emergence of 'new' diseases such as HIV infection indicate a need for health care professionals who are flexible and able to respond to change.
- International perspectives on the provision of community care will also demand the preparation of a more responsive and informed nurse in the future.

These influences have affected, and in many cases confirmed, the status of health care professionals within the context of a multidisciplinary team of specialist health care practitioners. Their work has also been directed by the advent of evidence-based practice, which has placed demands for new competencies amongst the work force, with an emphasis on research, therapeutic skills and care management. The challenges that these changes present for health service staff are summarised in the following quotation:

> The changes offer great opportunities – which must be carefully weighed. The results should be a strategy that embodies a concept for the future, is reflected in training and development at all levels, and produces caring, positive nurses who can face a turbulent and uncertain future with confidence in themselves and their values. (Department of Health, 1994, p. 23)

A BRIEF REVIEW OF THE LITERATURE ON STRESS AND COPING CAPACITY

In this section an overview of key concepts and issues arising from the literature is presented in so far as it forms the basis for discussion and understanding of the needs of staff experiencing new and challenging roles in what may be described for most as 'unfamiliar surroundings'.

Bowers (1973) indicated that for any theory of stress to be considered, account had to be taken of external influences and how they interact and change a person's behaviour. Mischel (1973) argued that any theory of human behaviour had to take account of three perspectives of 'environmental determinants, person variables, and experiential factors, i.e. the individual's subjective interpretation of events' (p. 257). Basowitz (1955) confirmed the interactive nature and influence of stress:

> We should not consider stress as imposed upon the organism, but as its response to internal or external processes which reach those threshold levels that strain the physical and psychological integrative capacities to, or beyond, their limits. (p. 78)

Individual perceptions of stress appear to be essential in the degree to which each person interprets or anticipates that external influences or changes will affect their state of equilibrium. This implies that people respond to stress when they believe that their coping strategies no longer protect them from external influences in their environment. Bannister and Fransella (1980) illustrate this well:

> It implies that you are not reacting to the past as much as reaching out to the future; it implies that you check how much sense you have made of the world by seeing how well that 'sense' enables you to anticipate it; it implies that your personality is the way you go about making sense of the world. (p. 89)

Stress may also be associated with a person's inability to predict the future and as such may have its origins in the way in which people interpret the world; this implies that individuals constantly test out their role in society against the expectations of others and against their own sense of reality and past experiences.

Bowers (1973) and French, Rogers and Cobb (1974) suggest that when stress arises from the lack of a good fit between the individual and their environment a number of coping behaviours come into play. Individuals may attempt to master their environment and try to manipulate circumstances in order to reduce stress. In hospital settings this may be seen amongst staff who choose to adopt a task-oriented approach to care rather than a person-centred approach.

Lazarus (1976) suggests that the two main coping behaviours utilized during stress are problem solving and emotional processing. In the former the individual will employ coping behaviours that they believe will lead to a positive outcome; in the latter the individual engages in the process of *cognitive reshaping* in an attempt to alter and lower their perception of stress or danger and thereafter cope more positively. Baley (1983) suggests that defence mechanisms are most important:

> Defence mechanisms are ways of coping. ... Short term denial to alleviate anxiety may help the nurse to carry on with nursing. Similarly, intellectualising the approach of surgery may be of some coping efficacy to surgeons and theatre nurses. Other defence mechanisms such as the employment of suppression, and detachment, may make 'space' for the health professional to mobilise more open forms of problem solving when emotional expression as a means of coping with stress is inappropriate. (p. 98)

In the work place, stress is common and accounts for many days of lost productivity. Personal perceptions of stress may be influenced by a variety of factors such as:

- Workload (overload and underload) (Margolis, 1974).
- Physiological strain (French *et al.*, 1965).
- Shift rotation (Selye, 1976).
- Role ambiguity (Khan *et al.*, 1964).
- Role conflict (Caplan and Jones, 1975).
- Responsibility (Wardwell, 1984).
- Relationships at work (Cooper and Marshall, 1987; Minzberg, 1973).
- Career development (Hingley and Cooper, 1983; Morris, 1975).
- Work–home interface (Beattie and Darlington, 1974; Gowler and Legge, 1975).

In 1988 the Health Education Authority published a report on stress in the public sector. They identified that health care professionals work in one of the most stressful professions:

> The nurse's role is … implicitly and chiefly one of handling stress. She is a focus for the stress of the patient, relatives and doctor, as well as her own. (Marshall, 1989)

They defined stress as 'an excess of demands on an individual beyond their ability to cope'. In their chapter on stress in nursing the authors confirmed that the main variables involved in the perception of stress included the leadership and management style of bosses, economic factors, conflict and ambiguity, public and social attitudes, client problems, training issues, interpersonal relationships, and matters relating to the organizational context of work.

It is also important to note that the effects of stress may be potentially damaging, as the following quotation from Holland (1987) suggests:

> The effects of stress are damaging both to the individual nurse, her relationships with colleagues, and ultimately, to the quality of care she helps to provide for patients and clients. We owe it to ourselves and others to gain insight into our existing coping strategies, to adapt and to improve upon them, and so develop a whole range of approaches to managing it more effectively. (p. 47)

LINKING THEORY AND PRACTICE – THE CHANGING CONTEXT OF CARE

Dunham (1978) noted that insecurity and unpredictability are major causes of stress in human services (p. 18). Reorganization, role ambiguity, and communication difficulties were also regarded as significant. He found that staff who reported lack of liaison with managers often had feelings of not being part of the system' (p. 19). This in turn might lead to a lack of commitment to the work of the organization:

> The barriers of effective inter-professional communication and co-operation with workers who are based outside the institution are caused by differences in professional experience ... we suffer from 'professional blindness'. (p. 19)

Dunham felt that, in order to overcome feelings of stress, staff should be encouraged to identify their own support systems and to develop a 'sense of belonging' by encouraging better interprofessional communications and supportive group networks.

Closely associated with stress and burnout is the experience of guilt that many staff appear to experience as a result of their increasing disengagement from their clients. Todd and Robinson (1989) argued that staff tend to act on impulse when under stress and tend to work more and more hours in order to accomplish their tasks. In time this approach results in fatigue and mistakes in their practical tasks, which in turn add to their feelings of guilt (p. 11). Walker found that health care professionals work under external pressure, which is a combination of public opinion and government policy, which are often in conflict over the availability of resources. In failing to cope with the sheer volume of work, the professional's identity may be shattered as they strive to provide the quality of care that they believe should be provided and yet fail to meet their objectives due to manpower deficiencies. Rather than blame their failures on the organization, many staff appear to assume direct ownership of the problem themselves, which in turn may lead to feelings of deep personal hurt.

The implications of stress and burnout for the caring professions are clear. There is a need to identify that services care for employees who provide direct care services to clients in demanding and continuous circumstances. According to Bailey (1988) it should be possible to ameliorate and prevent the effects of burnout for staff. The following quotation from Bailey (1988) summarizes the main issues to be considered:

> Underlying these premises is the fundamental assumption that to care more effectively for clients we must first of all begin to provide organisational initiatives which support the health and performance of those who deliver front-line health care services. ... Stress will not go away: some degree of stress is always essential for human health and performance. However, its potential lies in its promise to better manage, reduce and even avoid the exhaustion of personal resources consumed in the course of human helping. (p. 7)

STRESS AND SOCIAL CHANGE

One of the most important features of the NHS has been its stability as an organization. As such it has provided its employees with relatively stable work patterns. Cope (1984) acknowledges that this may be fine in an unchanging world but in the real world staff must adapt to organizational changes if they are to survive:

> Changes to organisations involve changing their working practices and procedures, and so require individuals to do things differently. 'Change' comes down eventually to getting people to do things in a new way. Sometimes when this concern is central to people's conceptions of themselves as persons this is extremely difficult to do. (p. 165)

This latter point is particularly true when related to staff working in the long-stay hospital services. Many staff working in these settings have been forced to change their work patterns as a result of social change. Staff in mental health and learning disability hospitals, for example, have been encouraged to seek new work opportunities in the community as the Government implements its 'care in the community' policy for long-stay client groups. For some of those nurses who were familiar with hospital-based routines the question of personal choice and control over where they work may not be an option. Such situations may lead to feelings of 'loss of control' or 'powerlessness' amongst the work force and may have a bearing on the extent to which health care professionals own or accept the changes imposed upon them. Mithaug and Hanawalt (1978) confirm:

> One should never assume that a choice has been made because the person has acted in a situation in which choice is permitted. (p. 155)

The shift in attitudes required to realize the philosophy of work in community services for many nurses in the long-stay sector may combine with new working patterns and service conditions to create new challenges and career opportunities for the work force. However, these new challenges may be perceived as threats in the first instance as staff strive to find the right balance between tolerance and firmness during the first few months of their new jobs.

THE NATURE OF STRESS AT WORK

Changes in the context of care (such as hospital closures or changes in routine) require staff to readjust their attitudes and work practices. Such changes demand that staff have to learn how to function in multidisciplinary teams and acquire new skills in presenting themselves as equal professionals alongside more 'experienced' peers.

Changing organizational systems also require health care professionals to exercise their own discretionary responsibility and to work with constantly changing situations which were not always tested or for which guiding rules do not appear to exist. One such example is the emergence of community-based residential care in the private sector, where relatively few tested support systems exist for staff.

Changes in workplace or routine may also demand that staff apply personal discretion, initiative, and judgement (skills that may be difficult for some staff to develop if they have been conditioned in the past to work within service systems where all decisions were sanctioned by line managers). In contrast, changes inherent in the new health care agenda now require staff to exercise their own discretion and to work with constantly changing situations for which rules may not have been prepared to guide them. This may result in stress for staff who may consider that their new roles are more ambiguous than those previously performed in traditional settings (such as long-stay hospitals). This calls for a constant evaluation of approach and for the calculation of risks.

In order to respond to changing care contexts managers are required to examine the effectiveness (and appropriateness) of staff support systems. Operational policies and staff development procedures will require revision in order to determine the standards of performance that should be expected from staff, and these in turn should facilitate the work force's effective contribution to the work of the changing organization. An examination of the appropriateness of existing policies and procedures should also accompany any organizational review to ensure that they are 'fit for the purpose' of the new work culture and philosophy. Failure to review such policies may instil conflict with the philosophy of the new order and present staff with both role conflict and ambiguity.

Staff will also demand that their employers provide them with a clear vision of the future, flexible access to staff development and counselling support, and effective feedback from managers. Personal training plans and effective communication networks should also be provided for staff.

MANAGERIAL COMPETENCE FOR PRACTICE

Contemporary health service structures require that clear organizational goals, aims, and objectives are set for each part of the service. Each component of the organization must therefore have a clear idea of what its business is and how it is going to translate its goals and objectives into operational practice.

The first principle should be for each organization to identify its business statement and to publish its aims and objectives, which must be defined in quantifiable and measurable terms. The degree to which each member of the organization shares in the beliefs expounded by senior managers must also be underpinned by processes that ensure that each staff member knows the role and contribution that they will be expected to play in achieving the organization's purpose, role, and function. Organizations should define each employee's scope of decision making, authority, and responsibility.

Once the organization has established its purpose and the extent of its range of business, it will need to ensure that it employs a skilled and competent work force to operationalize its objectives. In human care services this will require an understanding of the needs of the consumer or client group and the skills that will be required to meet their needs. The skills that will be required from the work force must be stated in terms of defined employment-led competencies; employers will need to ensure that systems are available to provide in-service training and continuing education for the work force in order to update, maintain, and motivate their staff and their skills to meet the ever changing demands of service users. Operational policies should be published within which the philosophy and values of the service are clearly described in measurable terms.

In order to ensure that staff provide effective care to their clients they must ensure that they are effectively supervised in all areas of their practice and keep in touch with the aims and objectives of senior managers. There are many ways of achieving this objective; perhaps the most successful has been the provision of clinical supervision and positive feedback from line managers. Clinical supervision is currently being introduced by the health service for staff, with the aim of providing them with a framework within which to receive positive feedback on their performance and to share their own perceptions of how well they are doing within the organization.

Effectiveness of service delivery will also depend on the motivation, commitment, and skills of staff, who will require personal leadership from their managers. Consequently all staff should be encouraged and empowered to set their own goals and targets through staff supervision and staff development performance review processes.

In order to achieve such aims and objectives all managers should provide firm guidance and support to staff to ensure that consistency of service delivery is achieved throughout their service. This may be facilitated through the setting of quality assurance targets and objectives in each person's annual review of performance, which in turn should lead to the publication of detailed plans for achieving high quality services. To do this staff will require:

- Commitment to providing the best possible service.
- Reinforcement of their individual contribution.
- The continuing development of team work throughout the organization.
- Encouragement of individual creativity and innovation within the context of clearly defined and agreed objectives.

Managers should therefore accept that change requires strategic management. Staff must be helped to move from a 'coping' style of management to one of 'confronting' (Davies, 1992). In her work on management styles in health care, Davies reported that many nursing staff had acquired a 'coping' style of management in response to many years of being disempowered by their managers and medical peers. Davies suggested that this style of working leads staff to accept less than favourable work conditions and to minimize the amount of challenge that they presented to their superiors. The 'coping manager' focuses her work on the immediate tasks to be accomplished and rarely succeeds in engaging in forward planning or strategic thinking. This leadership style is also characterized by feelings of low positive self-regard and status. Low expectations of management work to simplify the tasks of operational management, which in turn tends to encourage a task-oriented approach to care provision.

Davies suggests that one of the reasons why nurses tend to accept this style of management is that it seen by administrators and doctors as being a 'feminine' method of coping. Davies also notes in her work that this is due not so much to attribution to gender, but to the fact that the workplace is often structured around the working patterns of men and to the failure of many nurses (and other female health professionals) to articulate accurately the rationale for their practice.

Staff who adopt a coping style of management tend to suppress their frustrations and concerns and as result experience low morale, burnout, and low self-esteem. They may become introspective (within their professional group) and reduce opportunities for 'outsiders' (including managers) to understand the actual realities of their work practice and contribution to the work of the organization. By failing to advertise their contribution they convey a 'low level of intelligibility' to outsiders. This situation Davies refers to as 'a vicious circle of management'.

Conversely Davies (1992) notes that staff who articulate their knowledge base and demonstrate pride in the contribution that they and their profession make to the organization's business strengthen their position and gain respect and credibility as a result (rather than praise as is found with the coping style of management explained above). Such staff gain respect from their managers and engage in healthy debate and negotiation regarding work conditions and decision making. In return Davies believes that staff experience lower levels of stress, confidence, group cohesiveness, and higher morale and self-esteem. This approach to management Davies refers to as 'a virtuous circle of management' which provides staff and managers with the opportunity to acquire 'a growing understanding of issues' that concerns all levels of the organization.

If Davies' explanation is to be accepted then it would appear that any organizational review should encompass the challenge of examining the very infrastructure that shapes it, with the aim of encouraging transparency, mutual respect and dialogue between managers and employees.

IMPLEMENTING A COMPETENT WORKPLACE

Staff confronting change are challenged to maintain their professional credibility and to offer a genuine and responsive service to the public. A major investment is therefore required to facilitate the process of change and to provide a work force that is skilled and competent to meet the changing demands of technology, as well as the aim of meeting consumer requirements. There is also a growing awareness of the need to implement management support systems that are responsive to the needs of the work force.

David Pottage (1990), writing in response to the effects that change has on staff effectiveness, has introduced the concept of the 'competent workplace'. Pottage suggests that in order for organizations to demonstrate efficiency and effectiveness they have to transfer their 'mission' to the work force and examine the extent to which the workplace empowers workers to be creative and competent. He asks several key questions:

- How is the actuality of day to day work conveyed from front line workers to other parts of the organization?
- What mechanisms are in place for utilizing this information for operational and planning purposes?
- What are the means available for identifying and utilizing the skills of existing employees?
- How useful are the current profiles of staff members and facilities?
- To what extent are front line workers involved in service development activity?
- What is the nature of and extent of support offered to front line workers?
- How is monitoring and evaluation of operational activity currently undertaken, and, if it is, are explicit quality outcome criteria prescribed?

It is suggested that if organizations treat these questions seriously then the work force will be empowered to contribute efficiently and effectively to the work of the service. The success of any organization will therefore depend upon the way in which it responds to the needs of its staff. Staff in turn will interpret the value attributed to them by their superiors through an interpretation of the extent to which they perceive that their managers are listening to them and supporting them. Staff will also feel empowered if they are in receipt of information about the organization and if they are involved in decisions that will affect their future.

If staff are to feel genuinely empowered to contribute to the work of the organization they will require access to the decision-making process. Staff should, for example, develop their own policies and procedures rather than managers imposing restrictive policies on front line workers without consideration of the impact that these might have on reducing workplace efficiency and staff morale/ownership. Service quality will depend upon the extent to which staff are enabled to be creative and innovative. Service quality therefore depends upon empowerment of the work force; this requires that the organizational culture should encourage self-reflection and critical analysis of work performance by the work force itself. It will then be possible to reinforce the need for workers to review their own practices in order to move forward in response to external changes and demands.

Often, however, the reality is that centralized rules are imposed by managers with the result that individual staff empowerment opportunities are lost. Staff, willing to accept the challenge of change, may also find that the effect of a rigid rule-governed organizational culture results in major personal dilemmas. They may be encouraged to accept personal responsibility for their actions and yet be chastised for engaging in innovative practices. Staff faced with such dilemmas may experience considerable stress, which may cause concern as they engage in new roles. The following quotation from Charlotte Towle provides an illustration of these issues:

When an individual is insecure and when he is unable to master his environment, when he is not equipped to meet the changing demand of a situation he falls back on automatic behaviour as a source of security. Therefore, as the individual gains basic security in a work situation he will have less dependency on habitual ways and should move into a more flexible meeting of the varying aspects of the complex total of his job. Routines, regulations and fixed procedures constitute the medium for automatic behaviour in the social agency setting. Perhaps some of us have known the administrator, who, likewise, when he is insecure in his leadership or has little to bring to his staff in knowledge and certain professional skills, becomes anxiously engaged in drafting and re-drafting forms, procedures and checking up on his staff in relation to them. (Towle, 1957, p. 23)

CARING FOR THE CARER'S NEEDS

It is suggested that many health care workers feel swept along in a tide of irreversible change. The anxiety and stress arising from this organizational upheaval may be seen to cause the work force to adopt resilient attitudes and uncompromising values. However, given appropriate and responsive support, workers may adjust well to change and continue to provide a valuable contribution to the care of their clients.

The challenge now facing the health service implies that there will be a need to create a new multidisciplinary approach to leading and managing services within a climate characterized by increasing complexity, continual change, higher expectations from the consumer, and considerable political pressure. In order to compete with such demands it is suggested that full use will need to be made of all health care professionals as a major resource for the future. The challenge is therefore twofold:

• To release initiative, creativity, and commitment from the work force.
• To integrate people's agreed contributions towards agreed goals and philosophies of care.

The creation and maintenance of positive leadership in health care services requires that the conditions are created to ensure that these challenges are faced and that the work force is empowered to assume discretionary responsibility for personal practice in a variety of care settings, thus leading to an enriched standard of life for clients/patients.

In order to achieve these aims it is suggested that the following measures will be required in order to relieve stress in the workplace:

• Well defined systems, leadership, and accountability.
• Secure relationships between peers, managers, and members of the multidisciplinary team.

- Opportunities to be listened to in order to influence policy makers.
- Acceptance of the skilled contribution that staff are able to make (and will continue to make) to new services.
- Access to new relevant learning opportunities.
- Maintenance of a high level of self-esteem and appreciation for a 'job well done'.
- Design and publication of operational policies for the service, including clearly defined standards of expected practice and performance.
- Consistent feedback on performance from managers.
- Personal involvement in the evaluation and monitoring of service accomplishments.
- Reassurance of continuing resource provision for the effective delivery of effective care.
- Freedom from threat and the promise of job security.

Developing such a climate for leadership in health care services may provide staff with a more effective and responsive support network, which may ultimately lead to a major shift in the organizational culture within which local services are provided. For staff the realization that managers are prepared to change and to respond to the needs of the work force in a preventative way may lead to a reduction in the stress levels that they perceive to exist in their workplace.

Staff will also need to develop trust in their managers and to develop a partnership with them based on mutual respect and honesty. Staff and managers will also need to believe in each other and to acquire some degree of cohesion between their respective agendas in order to maintain the systems of care that all members of the organization are aiming to implement together. In order to empower staff their managers should provide:

- Clear information.
- Guidance and support during the transition period.
- Reassurance that skills and competencies will be valued in the new service (and a clear career pathway).
- Clear definition of role expectations.
- Procedures to monitor and evaluate the quality of the service.
- Assurance that adequate financial resources will be made available to support the new service.
- Responsive staff development and education strategies.
- Responsive management systems.
- Regular feedback on performance.
- The introduction of coping strategies to reduce the potential incidence of stress following the implementation of change (for example access to independent staff counselling services, mentors, and preceptors).

CONCLUSION

It is essential to affirm the principle that there are many advantages to maintaining a high standard of staff morale: a more contented staff means a lower turnover of staff, higher standards of care and an enhanced quality of life for the people they care for. It is the author's overwhelming conclusion that in this health and cost conscious age, the health and social care systems in Britain can no longer afford to ignore the issue of staff support for its many health care professionals.

This chapter ends with a challenge encapsulated in the words of Charles Handy:

> Continuous change requires discontinuous thinking. If the new way of things is going to be different from the old, not just an improvement on it, then we shall need to look at everything in a new way.
>
> These new ways need a new language to describe them. A language of federations and networks of alliances and influences: that language requires us to learn new habits, to live with more uncertainty but more creativity. (Charles Handy, 1989, p. 87).

REFERENCES

Bailey, R. (1988) Burnt-out – counselling and the health care professions. *J. Health Care Management*, **3** (1), 5–8.

Baley, M. (1983) *Nursing and Social Change*, Heinemann, London.

Bannister, D. and Fransella, F. (1980) *Inquiring Man*, Penguin, Harmondsworth.

Basowitz, H. *et al.* (1955) *Anxiety and Stress*, McGraw-Hill, New York.

Beattie, R.T. and Darlington, T.G. (1974) *The Management Threshold*, OPN, 11, British Institute of Management Paper, London.

Bowers, K.S. (1973) Situationalism in psychology: an analysis and critique. *Psychological Review*, **80**, 307–35.

Caplan, R.D. and Jones, K.W. (1975) Organisational stress and individual strain: a social-psychological study of risk factors in administrators. Unpublished PhD thesis, University of Michigan.

Cooper, C.L. and Marshall, J. (1987) *Understanding Executive Stress*, Macmillan, London.

Cope, D. (1984) Changing health care organisations, in *Understanding Nurses* (ed. S. Skevington), John Wiley, New York.

Davies, C. (1992) Gender, history and management style in nursing: towards a theoretical analysis, in *Gender and Bureaucracy*, (eds M. Savage and A. Witz), Blackwell, Oxford.

Department of Health (1992) *The Patient's Charter*, HMSO, London.

Department of Health (1994) *The Challenges for Nursing and Midwifery in the 21st Century – 'The Heathrow Report'*, HMSO, London.

Dunham, J. (1978) Staff stress in residential work. *Social Work Today*, **9** (45), 18–20.

French, J.P.R. *et al.* (1965) Workload of university professors. Unpublished research report, University of Michigan.

French, J.P.R., Rogers, W. and Cobb, S. (1974) A model of person–environment fit, in *Coping and Adaptation*, (eds D.A. Hamburgh and G.E. Adams), Basic Books, New York.

Gowler, D. and Legge, K. (1975) *Managerial Stress*, Gower Press, Epping.

Handy, C (1989) *The Age of Unreason*, Hutchinson, London.

Health Education Authority (1988) *Stress in the Public Sector – Nurses, Police, Social workers and Teachers*, HEA, London.

Hingley, P. and Cooper, C.L. (1983) The others at the top: the personality characteristics of key change agents. *New Society*, October.

Holland, S. (1987) Stress in nursing – what does stress do to you? *Nursing Times*, **83** (30), 44–7.

Khan, R.L. *et al.* (1964) *Organisational Stress*, John Wiley, New York.

Lazarus, R.S. (1976) *Patterns of Adjustment*, McGraw-Hill, New York.

Margolis, B.L. (1974) Work and the health of man, in *Work and the Quality of Life* (ed. P. O'Toole), MIT Press, Cambridge, Mass.

Marshall, R. (1989) Blood and gore. *The Psychologist*, **2** (3), 115–17. BPS. London.

Minzberg, H. (1973) *The Nature of Managerial Work*, Harper & Row, New York.

Mischel, W. (1973) Towards a cognitive social learning reconceptualisation of personality. *Psychological Review*, **80**, 252–83.

Mithaug, D.E. and Hanawalt, D.A. (1978) The validation of procedures to assess pre-vocational task preferences in retarded adults. *Journal of Applied Behavioural Analysis*, **1**, 153–62.

Morris, J. (1975) Managerial stress and the 'cross of relationships', in *Managerial Stress* (eds D. Gowler and K. Legge), Gower Press, Epping.

Pottage, D. (1990) The competent workplace – making NVQ work for social care. Unpublished report, Department of Philosophy, University of Manchester.

Selye, H. (1976) *The Stress of Life*, McGraw-Hill, New York.

Todd, C. and Robinson, G. (1989) *Twelve versus eight hour shifts: job satisfaction of nurses and quality of care provided*. Centre for Applied Health Studies, University of Ulster, Coleraine, UK.

Towle, C (1957) *Common Human Needs*, revised edn, National Association of Social Workers, USA.

Wardwell, J. (1984) *Planning for people: developing a local service for people with a mental handicap*, King's Fund, London.

<table>
<tr><td>8</td><td># Stress in nursing and health visiting: the potential of clinical supervision</td></tr>
</table>

| 8 | # Stress in nursing and health visiting: the potential of clinical supervision |

Tony Butterworth

PROGRESS IN CLINICAL SUPERVISION

Clinical supervision and its delivery is developing apace in nursing and midwifery in the United Kingdom. It appears to be shaping into 'ideal types' (Houston 1990). One to one sessions with a supervisor from the same discipline are reported (Dewing 1994). One to one peer supervision has also been reported (Semperingham 1994), but interestingly has also been criticized as being the most likely method to be open to difficulty because of the dangers of slipping into a consensus collusion (Faugier and Butterworth 1994). Peer group supervision has found favour particularly among district nurses and health visitors (Johnson 1995). While networking supervision is reportedly used by nurse specialists in such areas as HIV/AIDS care and Macmillan nursing there appear to be no reported data. There has been a view that the cost consequences of implementing clinical supervision may hinder its implementation; however, such little evidence as there is shows the consequences to be less significant than many might suppose (Dudley and Butterworth 1994).

There is evidence of an 'ideological shift' as the territory relating to clinical supervision has become more clear and ideas progress (Brocklehurst, 1994). It may be evidence of practice developing around clinical supervision and the influences of newly developing health care services which are changing the focus of the debate. Inevitably the debate will benefit as further changes are identified in the reporting of data.

The introduction of the Code of Professional Conduct (UKCC, 1986), has significance when one considers autonomy and accountability in practice within the reduced professional support mechanisms in flattened hierarchies. Clinical supervision has been seen to provide a useful framework for the Department of Health for developing and supporting those in practice and has consequently had the support of strategic planning from the Chief Nursing Officer (CNO) and others. The Chief Nursing Officer (CNO) recommended in the policy plan *Vision for the Future* (Department of Health, 1993) that 'the concept of clinical supervision should be further explored and developed. Discussions should be held at a local and national level on the range and appropriateness of models of clinical supervision and a report made available to the professions …' The report *Clinical Supervision: A Position Paper* (Faugier and Butterworth, 1994) was produced the following year and widely distributed to the profession by the Department of Health. In an accompanying letter the CNO stated, 'I have no doubt as to the value of clinical supervision and consider it to be fundamental to safeguarding standards, the development of professional expertise and the delivery of care' (Department of Health, 1994a,b). The recent Allitt Inquiry (HMSO, 1994) has also crystallized a number of concerns about the supervision of safe and accountable practice. It has been argued that clinical supervision can help to sustain and develop safe and accountable practice (Butterworth and Faugier, 1994). It was also commonly agreed and endorsed by participants in a Delphi survey of optimum practice (Butterworth and Bishop, 1995) that a system should be in place which empowers practitioners and protects patients by regulation and the promotion of good practice.

In a further drive from the Department of Health, the CNO, in collaboration with the *Nursing Times*, raised the profile of clinical supervision with practising nurses and health visitors (Bishop 1994) and developed, in conjunction with the Trust Nurse Executives a three-point plan in which a national workshop for Trust Nurse Executives, a national conference for the profession, and a multi-site evaluation research project were proposed. The two conferences were held and have been reported upon (Department of Health, 1994b, 1995a) and the multi-site evaluation project was completed in 1996–97.

In its most recent update on work by the professions (Department of Health, 1995b), commenting on progress on Target 10 from *Vision for the Future*, the NHS Executive suggests that 'National initiatives which lead to improved clinical supervision, developing professional consensus on the key elements of clinical supervision and ensuring consistency with UKCC guidance should inform developments at local level. Improved understanding of the cost benefits of clinical supervision will need to be developed between purchasers and providers and a nurse or health visitor could be seconded to carry out the necessary developmental work.'

The United Kingdom Central Council for Nursing, Health Visiting, and Midwifery (1993) has suggested a model for the continuum of practice in which 'practitioners have no end point in their need to maintain and develop standards of practice'. A definitive position statement on clinical supervision for nursing and health visiting has now been issued (UKCC, 1996).

EVALUATING CLINICAL SUPERVISION

Any attempt at evaluating clinical supervision is fraught with difficulty. A broad methodological framework using both qualitative and quantitative approaches is likely to be the most productive means to finding answers.

'Ideal' research answers will be those in which clinical supervision is shown to have an impact on patient outcome; however, the development of clinical supervision is such that in many services it is likely to be so immature an activity as to make it impossible to focus on patient change as an indicator for evaluation. The pressures to take this approach are considerable as 'evidence based practice' becomes the gold standard of our clinical activity. However, so early in its development a measured and wide-ranging approach is likely to produce more satisfactory and reliable results.

There is considerable merit in finding the impact of clinical supervision on the well-being of staff given the simple but obvious truism that 'happy nurse equals happy patient'. At a more fundamental level, recent anecdotal reports of an unhappy work force and unwillingness of people to enter the nursing and medical professions must be investigated thoroughly if these depressing trends are to be reversed. Staff well-being and psychological health are fundamental to these matters and it is possible that clinical supervision will impact on them.

It is becoming possible to identify some evaluation techniques that can assist practitioners, purchasers, and providers to assess the usefulness of clinical supervision and its impact on the work force. The following matters are seen as important in auditing and monitoring clinical supervision: (i) defining and agreeing the agencies' ground rules; (ii) devising and monitoring the agencies' plans for implementing and sustaining clinical supervision; (iii) looking at the provision of education and development; (iv) monitoring and maintaining lists of supervisors; (v) deciding on a mechanism for evaluation (Butterworth and Faugier, 1994).

Trust Nurse Executives (Department of Health, 1994b) have suggested that it may be possible to audit clinical supervision through existing mechanisms, such as: rates of sickness and absence, staff satisfaction scales, numbers of patient complaints, retention and recruitment of staff, and critical incident maps. However, it is recognized that more sophisticated tools must be developed and a national study is now underway to try and develop this work further.

At a Department of Health funded workshop, evaluation and clinical supervision were debated at length. In a positional paper (now reprinted as an appendix to the printed conference proceedings of a major national conference in the West Midlands (Department of Health, 1995a)) a number of working principles were suggested and are re-presented here. Few, if any, have yet been tested in the context of clinical supervision for nurses and health visitors.

Using the component elements of clinical supervision as suggested by Proctor (1992) it is possible to offer the first steps in an evaluation strategy. These first steps seek to evaluate the core principle of clinical supervision, that of supporting staff. Progressively, work should also seek to link clinical supervision to clinical outcomes.

The normative component

The normative component is that which addresses those issues of practice that relate to quality control and the demands of the organization. By examining data already gathered for general information purposes it is likely that one will find data relating to the value of clinical supervision from clinical audit, staff satisfaction scales, rates of sickness/absence, and numbers of patient complaints. Assessment tools exist that might further inform this process, for example the Minnesota Job Satisfaction Scale (Cooper, Sloan and Williams, 1988). This is a 20 item questionnaire that was developed in the USA based on Herzberg's theory of work motivation. Items are rated on a five-point scale from 1 = 'very dissatisfied' to 5 = 'very satisfied.' Three scores are obtained. Intrinsic satisfaction (12 items) reflects a person's degree of contentment with the job itself in terms of achievement, recognition, or responsibility. Extrinsic satisfaction (six items) looks at contentment with factors such as salary, status, security, and supervision. Both these are combined with an additional two items to give a total job satisfaction score.

The restorative component

The restorative component of clinical supervision relates to the supportive help that must be available for professionals working constantly with stress and distress. Clinical supervision is seen by some as a proactive, protective device to assist coping, which has more value than waiting for reactive solutions to damage already done to the work force. There are a number of measures available that have been used successfully and a selection are presented here.

NURSE STRESS INDEX (HARRIS, 1989)

This 30 item questionnaire was developed following extensive piloting work involving over 300 nurses. From an initial index of 52 items a short form of 30 items was constructed. This comprises six factors with five questions in each section. The areas covered are: managing the workload, parts 1 and 2; organizational support and involvement; dealing with patients and relatives; home–work conflict; confidence and competence in role. The questionnaire was subsequently administered to 470 nurses.

CLAYBURY CPN STRESS QUESTIONNAIRE (REVISED) (BROWN ET AL., 1995)

This 48 item scale was developed to assess stress in community mental health nurses. Staff are asked to rate a list of stressors on a five-point scale: 0 = 'this activity causes me no stress', to 4 = 'I feel extremely stressed by this activity'. It is a specific measure of stress for community mental health nurses, though at least two other researchers have modified it slightly for use with health visitors.

GOODMAYES PSYCHIATRIC STRESS QUESTIONNAIRE (DEVILLIERS ET AL., 1995)

This is a recently developed 30 item measure of stress among ward-based mental health nurses. Factor analysis suggested a five-factor solution. These were: clinical demand; organization and management; staffing concerns; future issues; job satisfaction. The questionnaire is rated in the same way as the CPN Stress Questionnaire.

MASLACH BURNOUT INVENTORY (MASLACH AND JACKSON, 1986)

This is a measure of 'occupational burnout syndrome'. It has 22 items that are scored on a frequency of occurrence basis. Items cover an individual's feelings or attitudes towards their work. The questionnaire has three independent subscales: emotional exhaustion (9 items), depersonalization (5 items), and personal accomplishment (8 items). It is probably the most widely used assessment in the worldwide nursing stress literature.

GENERAL HEALTH QUESTIONNAIRE (GHQ-28) (GOLDBERG AND WILLIAMS, 1988)

A 28 item questionnaire that measures an individual's level of psychological distress. It has four formats: 60, 30, 28, and 12 item forms. The most recent version of the manual has been expanded to incorporate the rapidly growing worldwide literature on this measure. The 28 item form has four subscales: somatic symptoms; anxiety and insomnia; social dysfunction; severe depression. In non-clinical samples, the GHQ total score is the most important score obtained from the scale.

COOPER COPING SKILLS QUESTIONNAIRE (COOPER, SLOAN AND WILLIAMS, 1988)

This 28 item questionnaire is part of the Occupational Stress Indicator. It asks participants how often they utilize specific coping strategies, on a six-point scale from 1 = 'never used by me', to 6 = 'very extensively used by me'. The scale has six subscales: social support; task strategies; logic; home and work relationship; time; involvement.

The formative component

The formative component of clinical supervision relates to the educative process of developing skills. In this domain, nurses and health visitors are seen to be developing life-long learning through the opportunity that clinical supervision provides them to observe and reflect upon their practice and the skills needed to carry it out.

Collectively, evaluation might be done by assessing the progress of supervisees through the normal processes of continuous education audit, individual performance review, and development of specialist skills in new methods of service delivery.

At an individual level, evaluation relating to observed performance means that the supervisor might need access to actual data in the form of observations, audiotape recordings, or videotape recordings of clinical practice. Part of the usefulness of this data relates to the ongoing work of the supervisor and supervisee in making theory-based links to practice problems. It can also provide a means to having material that can be rated through some more structured means for those seeking to assess the capacity of the supervisee to demonstrate qualities in their work which show evidence of newly developed skills.

In summary, the formative component of clinical supervision might be carried out using: (i) Trust-wide educational audit; (ii) individual performance review; (iii) assessment of new skills in innovative service delivery; (iv) live supervision recorded on video or audio tape; (v) retrospective analysis of audiotape or videotape recordings; (vi) live or retrospective analysis of observation notes.

ESTABLISHING A MULTI-SITE EVALUATION PROJECT

While the nursing profession has been generally supportive of the implications of clinical supervision, practitioners and mangers alike have shown a proper concern that the investment in it would be reflected in benefits both to patients and to the work force. In March 1995 a Department of Health funded workshop on the use of selected assessment tools to evaluate the effectiveness of clinical supervision was organized and presented by the author and others. Following this a letter was sent from the NHS Nursing Directorate to every Trust Nurse Executive inviting them to tender for pump-priming funds to evaluate models of clinical supervision. Clear criteria had to be met in order that, as far as possible, like would be compared with like. From the enthusiastic responses 18 sites were selected which offered geographic spread and a wide variety of specialities. Additionally Scotland has agreed to follow a similar format, thus enlarging the study to 23 sites across two countries.

A research project proposal from the University of Manchester was presented to the Department of Health, suggesting a multi-site evaluation project with the following aims: (i) to give an informed view on assessment tools that can be used to report on the impact of clinical supervision; (ii) to report on the activities of selected experimental sites that have evaluated some elements of clinical supervision within a specified format. The proposal suggested using demographic data, organizational data, a series of measures, and selected interviews; the proposal was accepted and a project timetable developed.

Eighteen sites in England and five sites in Scotland were selected for a centrally funded evaluation project in which a prescribed number of evaluation exercises are followed. Three thousand pounds per site were made available for evaluation support over a nine-month period. The sites have the following characteristics:

(1) A named evaluation site coordinator. This person is a registered graduate nurse with some research experience and has sufficient management support to drive the programme successfully. The site coordinator obtains: (i) the required access to nurses, midwives, and health visitors; (ii) the necessary ethics committee approval to proceed; (iii) the required evaluation data within prescribed guidelines.

(2) Sites have to offer three sample cohorts: one that is involved in clinical supervision as supervisees (10 in total) and another matched group of 10 practitioners who are not involved in clinical supervision to act as controls (180 supervisees and 180 controls, $n = 360$). Up to ten supervisors will also be assessed at each site.

(3) The provision of clinical supervision for the 'active' group has to conform to certain characteristics, namely: (i) a written supervision contract must have been made between supervisors and supervisees; (ii) a defined time (not less than 45 minutes every four weeks) must have been allocated to clinical supervision in the 'active' group; (iii) the process of clinical supervision offered must be actively considering the 'normative', 'formative', and 'restorative' requirements of the supervisee.

(4) The capacity to administer a focused questionnaire to up to 10 supervisors at each site. Groups have been set up so that the following data can be gathered:

- Group A (a control group) – never exposed to clinical supervision but given measures twice in a nine-month period.
- Group B (the test group) – exposed to clinical supervision and given measures twice in a nine-month period.
- Group C (a nested group) – group A become a third group who after nine months are exposed to clinical supervision and are tested another nine months later.
- Group D (the clinical supervisors) – exposed to clinical supervision and given measures twice in a nine-month period.

Demographic data are gathered from each site on age, sex, grade, and other brief views on work, including self-assessments of health, sickness, and absence. Participants are given measures from standardized instruments. All measures are given twice in a nine-month period and will include: (i) the Minnesota Job Satisfaction Scale; (ii) the General Health Questionnaire;

(iii) the Maslach Burnout Inventory; (iv) the Cooper Coping Skills Questionnaire; and (v) the Harris Nurse Stress Index.

Selected participants are given the chance for individual expression through a taped interview at six sites; interviewees will include site coordinators and managers. The timetable for the project is: June/July 1995, data gathering; July/September 1995, data analysis; September/December 1996, interviews with selected participants; February 1996, second data collection; June 1996, report to the Department of Health.

STRESS, NURSING, AND HEALTH VISITING: SOME PRELIMINARY THOUGHTS ON CLINICAL SUPERVISION

At the time of writing this chapter, data from the national evaluation is insufficiently complete to offer firm views on the effect that clinical supervision may have on the stress levels of staff and their psychological well-being. However, some indicators are apparent that suggest that clinical supervision allows staff to reflect positively upon themselves and is greatly valued. In the survey, individuals and site coordinators have shown a high regard for the opportunity to talk about and reflect upon their practice. Through this it is widely believed that better and more confident practice is occurring.

Staff in nursing and health visiting are presented each day with complex situations by colleagues, relatives, and circumstances that cause them stress, distress, and anxiety. This inevitably takes its toll and any device that allows some alleviation of this must be positive and to their general advantage. Although clinical supervision is by no means an answer to the problems of working as a nurse or health visitor it appears to confer some benefits to demanding and often unpredictable work.

REFERENCES

Bishop, V. (1994) Clinical supervision; questionnaire results. *Research in Practice*, **90** (48), 40–2.

Brocklehurst, N.J. (1994) Developing a model of clinical supervision for community nursing; the case of district nurses and HIV disease. Unpublished MSc thesis, University of Manchester.

Brown, D., Leary, J., Carson, J. *et al.* (1995) Stress and the community mental health nurse: the development of a measure. *Journal of Psychiatric and Mental Health Nursing*, **2**, 1–5.

Butterworth, T. and Bishop, V. (1995) Identifying the characteristics of optimum practice: findings from a survey of practice experts in nursing, midwifery and health visiting. *Journal of Advanced Nursing*, **22**, 24–32.

Butterworth, T. and Faugier, J. (1994) *Clinical Supervision in Nursing, Midwifery and Health Visiting: A Briefing Paper*, School of Nursing Studies, University of Manchester.

Cooper, C., Sloan, S. and Williams, S. (1988) *The Occupational Stress Indicator*, NFER–Nelson, Windsor.

Department of Health (1993) *Vision for the Future*, Report of the Chief Nursing Officer, HMSO, London.

Department of Health (1994a) Clinical supervision for the nursing and health visiting professions. CNO. Letter 94 (5).

Department of Health (1994b) *Clinical Supervision: A Report of the Trust Nurse Executives Workshops*, (eds T. Butterworth and V. Bishop), NHS Executive.

Department of Health (1995a) *Clinical Supervision*, conference proceedings from a national workshop at the National Motorcycle Museum, NHS Executive.

Department of Health (1995b) *'Vision for the Future' Implementation and Evaluation 1995 and Beyond*, NHS Executive.

DeVilliers, N., Carson, J., Leary, J. *et al.* (1995) Stress in ward based mental health nurses: the development and piloting of a new measure.

Dewing, J. (1994) Report on Burford Community Hospital, in *Clinical Supervision in Practice* (ed. N. Kohner), King's Fund Centre BEBC, Dorset.

Dudley, M. and Butterworth, T. (1994) The costs and some benefits of clinical supervision: an initial exploration. *The International Journal of Psychiatric Nursing Research*, **1** (2), 34–40.

Faugier, J. and Butterworth, T. (1994) *Clinical Supervision: A Position Paper*, School of Nursing Studies, University of Manchester.

Goldberg, D. and Williams, P. (1988) *A Users Guide to the General Health Questionnaire*, NFER–Nelson, Windsor.

Harris, P. (1989) The nurse stress index. *Work and Stress* **3** (4), 335–46.

HMSO (1994) The Allitt Inquiry: Independent inquiry relating to deaths and injuries on the children's ward at Grantham and Kesteven General Hospital during the period February to April 1991. HMSO, London.

Houston, G. (1990) *Supervision and Counselling*, The Rochester Foundation. London.

Johnson, P. (1995) The community services view, in *Clinical Supervision*, conference proceedings, NHS Executive, August.

Maslach, C. and Jackson, S. (1986) *Maslach Burnout Inventory*, Consulting Psychologists Press, California.

Proctor, B. (1992) In *Supervision in the Helping Professions* (ed. P. Hawkins and R. Shoet), Open University Press, Milton Keynes.

Semperingham, J. (1994) Report on Eillen Skellern Three Ward, in *Clinical Supervision in Practice* (ed. N. Kohner) King's Fund Centre BEBC, Dorset.

United Kingdom Central Council (UKCC) (1986) *Code of Professional Conduct for the Nurse, Midwife and Health Visitor*, UKCC, London.

United Kingdom Central Council (1993) *Report on the Post-Registration Education and Practice Project*, UKCC, London.

United Kingdom Central Council (UKCC) (1996) *Position Statement on Clinical Supervision for Nursing and Health Visiting*, UKCC, London.

In-patient services for sick health care professionals

9

Sally Hardy*, Mike Gill and Catherine Adcock

The impact of occupational stress on health care workers and their clinical practice has been subject to much debate but little research. There are many aspects of working in the health care arena that are individually considered stressful (for example, long working hours, work overload, and lack of support) but there appears to be a reluctance to formulate the conclusion that caring for others should carry a government health warning.

This chapter and the project described represent an opportunity to understand further some of the particular difficulties encountered by health care workers who develop mental illness. The project was devised and carried out by members of a multidisciplinary team involved in setting up and running a service for health care workers with mental health problems in south London. Particular importance was placed on providing a service that was both competent, confidential, and away from the individuals' professional work environment. All of this amounted to a recognized need for a rigorous investigation into the implications of the work environment on the health and well-being of health care workers. In this chapter, we have concentrated on the qualitative data derived from semi-structured interviews of 12 health professionals and eight people in professions outside health care.

INTRODUCTION

Mental illness accounts for approximately 20 per cent of certified sickness (Waldegrave, 1991). Using this figure, it can be estimated that nearly 150,000 health employees are absent from work on any one day due to mental health prob-

* Contact for further information on the statistical analysis and details of this project, c/o the publisher.

lems. Eighty million working days are lost through mental illness per year, costing employers nearly £4 billion (Jenkins and Coney, 1992). Most people attribute their mental illness to their job or work-related stress (Cherry, 1978; Warr and Payne, 1988) and there is increasing evidence to indicate that health workers are amongst the greatest group at risk (Dolan, 1987; Tyler and Cushway, 1992; Caplan, 1994).

In August 1992, an in-patient unit was opened at the Bethlem and Maudsley NHS Trust. The unit aimed to provide a specialist service to health care workers suffering from mental health problems. Previously care for NHS employees had been on the basis of complementary arrangements with neighbouring health authorities.

Clinical experience indicated that patients suffered a wide range of acute and chronic mental health problems and in addition suffered from acute professional embarrassment. Patients found it difficult to own up to their problems and felt that the very nature of their work meant that seeking help equated with an inability to function properly as a health professional. This clinical evidence needed to be tested by comparison with the work experiences of other professional groups. The new service was still in its infancy, so research was needed to ensure the service was adequately meeting the needs of its patient group.

During the three years the service was in operation more than 200 health care workers were treated. The unit provided individual and group therapy and advocated the need for health workers to feel able to be the patient. The ward based its philosophy of care on the work of Jackson and Cawley (1992), who advocate a psychodynamic principle to the ward, with each individual having an influence on the therapeutic environment and treatment process. Over 94 per cent of all cases were successful in resulting in the patient being able to return to work.

IMPETUS FOR THE RESEARCH PROJECT

Clinical experience of providing care for health care workers over the three years the service was running suggested to us that patients failed to or were unable to seek help early on in their illness due to the nature of their profession. As a result they invariably required an urgent admission, often following a catastrophic event. If this were true, more work needed to be done to enable the service to meet the need for early intervention, resulting in brief hospital admissions and a smooth transition back to work.

Previous studies on occupational stress for health care workers rely on anecdotal evidence, do not attempt to standardize stress, and do not use controls (Caplan, 1994). The present study therefore attempted to use both standardized stress measures and a control group to explore the effect of occupational stress. The sample was taken from all first admissions to the Bethlem and Maudsley NHS Trust between August 1992 and August 1993. Controls were selected from contemporary admissions to other units in the hospital.

TRACKING DOWN THE EVIDENCE

Most literature concentrates on the medical profession (or 'sick doctors'). Specific work-related stress has been identified as heavy workload, the on-call system, dealing with death and dying, and lack of social and emotional support due to alienation from family and friends through long and antisocial working hours (Bailey, 1985). Within nursing, attention to stress at work has been mounting. Emotional upset is one area identified as stressful for those health workers involved in dealing with trauma, including paramedics and ambulance crew. Trauma can be met on a daily basis (Menzies-Lyth, 1989) but is also experienced in major disasters (e.g. the Marchioness pleasure cruise sinking on the Thames and the Clapham train crash). Many ambulance and nursing staff can all too readily recount with graphic detail the visions and emotions experienced during these times. A colleague working at Guy's Hospital casualty department said he worked that night on automatic pilot until the morning after, when he felt sick, faint, and totally overwhelmed as the images came home of just what some of the patients he had dealt with so calmly had experienced. This vision stayed with him for many months. Ambulance staff reported receiving little or no support or counselling, but were called off to another job minutes after pulling bodies from the wrecks. The same reports were given from the police and fire brigade. One policeman said, 'a leaflet was sent round asking if we wanted counselling and you had to tick a box saying yes or no – not very conducive to get you to recognize the value of counselling if that's their attitude'.

JOB STRESS IN THE WORKPLACE

Investigation has taken place into stress in the workplace. Particular attention has been paid to 'high risk' jobs, such as air traffic controllers, police, executives, and nurses (Cooper and Kelly, 1993). There has, however, been little research in the area of stress and its negative effect on mental health in relation to health care workers. What is the evidence to say that working in the health care setting is particularly stressful compared to other professions? Do health care workers fail to elicit help for their conditions and, if so, why? Both these important questions were major considerations of the project team.

Tyler and Cushway (1992) in their study of 72 hospital nurses identified work overload as having a particularly negative effect on health outcomes, measured from six different questionnaires. They described work overload as resulting from organizational changes and staff shortages. They also discussed negative coping styles adopted by nurses, but recognized the limitation of this statement. Clearly one person's coping style might be wholly inappropriate for another.

ATTITUDES AND JOB PERFORMANCE

The empirical evidence to support a relationship between one's attitude and job performance is limited. Historically, attitudes have been defined as the readiness to respond to a situation. Attitudes are hypothetical constructs (therefore inferred), resulting in the need for a particular method of measurement. Traditionally, attitudes are measured by self-reports of beliefs, feelings, and intentions. Attitude variance in a particular sample might be random but there is growing evidence that job attitudes vary systematically with the characteristics of the employee's position in the organization and their demographic background. Gibson (1966) suggests that the relationship depends upon the terms of the psychological contract between the employee and employer. If the cost of an absence (either in pay or in the legitimate procedure) were greater than the gain from the absence, absenteeism would not be a reasonable behaviour alternative. Job satisfaction remains only loosely related to absenteeism. However, not all empirical studies of job satisfaction take into consideration situation contingencies.

Job attitudes and job performance relationships only seem to occur in situations where job behaviour is primarily worker controlled. An employee's attitude may vary with their perception and evaluation of relevant events in their job situation. Workers who are dissatisfied with their job may respond in various ways. They can resign, go off sick, or file a grievance to try and change the situation. They can alter their job performance, and reduce the quantity of work produced. The quality of care provision is therefore loosely related to job satisfaction and stress. In other words, if a professional is feeling stressed they are not as able to care so effectively.

Owing to the non-specific nature of previously published literature, our research aims were focused on the effect of work-related stress on the mental health of health care workers, using the control group of other professionals as a means of comparing results and testing our hypothesis. The research aims were as follows:

(1) To determine whether health care workers (HCW) who develop mental illness remain in post and do not seek help because of the nature of their work.
(2) To determine the routes by which HCWs come to be referred to mental health services.
(3) To measure the time lapse between the first signs of mental illness and referral to the mental health services.
(4) To identify the proportion of HCWs who are able to return to work following mental illness.
(5) To assist in the development of a needs-led service for HCWs who suffer mental illness.

RESEARCH DESIGN

The project is a case control study comparing 20 first admission health care professionals with employment and responsibility matched controls drawn from other admissions to the Bethlem and Maudsley NHS Trust ($n = 40$). Comparisons were made for:

* Work record of the year preceding admission.
* Contact with the mental health care services.
* Involvement with work colleagues or occupational health departments.
* Perceived role of work-related stress in precipitating mental illness.

MEASURES

It was considered necessary to use both qualitative and quantitative measures in the study of stress. First there was the problem of obtaining an operational definition of stress and second the problem that obtaining empirical data in isolation does not allow consideration of the effect of individual responses to stress, as recognized in the Caplan (1994) project.

All cases were assessed using a semi-structured interview (designed by the authors), an anxiety stress questionnaire (House and Rizzo, 1972), a job satisfaction questionnaire (Brayfield and Ruth, 1951), a job role questionnaire (Beehr, Walsh and Taber, 1976), and a dysfunctional attitudes scale and visual analogue scales (designed by the authors).

A selection of matched controls was made from a list of all new admissions between August 1992 and August 1993 using employment criteria derived from salary range, years of training, and number of people under the person's supervision.

Data collection

Before any contact was made with participants, the hospital's ethical committee approved the project. Then, the 20 cases and 20 controls outlined previously were selected. Letters were sent to each consultant psychiatrist informing them of the research study aims and requesting their approval to contact their patients. Once consent was obtained from the consultants the 40 patients were sent consent and information letters plus a stamped addressed envelope for a rapid response. Once consent was received from the participants, another letter was sent, thanking them for responding and suggesting times and dates for interviews (with author CA). Additional correspondence confirmed the date and time of the interview. Interview rooms were booked in the out-patient department to ensure few interruptions and privacy for the duration of the interview, allowing some additional time for the participant to discuss any issues raised by the questionnaire.

Forty-four people were identified as possible candidates, of which 40 were contacted by post (four people could not be traced). The participants' addresses ranged from the inner and south London area to as far afield as Yorkshire.

We obtained 19 replies from written and telephone contact, with 21-non responses (approximately a 50 per cent response rate). The non-responders consisted of 13 people who failed to respond at all, two who had moved out of the country, three who were considered too unwell (one candidate's wife wrote to inform us of her husband's deteriorating mental and physical health; the other two were admitted to hospital in acute phases of mental and physical illness). There were two refusals and one deceased.

Participants were met and once again the purpose of the interview was explained and the procedure outlined, with an estimation of how long the interview would last. Interviews lasted approximately 1–2 hours. Coffee was provided and participants were consulted as to what they wished done with the confidential written material once the research was complete. Those participants who could not travel for a face to face interview were sent questionnaires and self-rating scales through the post, with additional instructions and a covering letter.

The semi-structured interview

The interviewer asked questions in an objective manner to avoid bias in responses and recorded the responses on a preformatted sheet. Adequate time was allowed for participants to expand on issues that were being discussed. Following the interview the participant was asked to complete five self-rating scales. On completion the participant was again thanked for their time and asked if they wished for a copy of the final report. Assistance was offered to cover travel expenses but this offer was not taken up by any of the volunteers.

RESULTS

Statistical data have yet to be completed. Owing to the limitations of the chapter and the nature of this book, results will concentrate on the qualitative data. The data presented here form the basis of issues to be explored in the discussion section.

Qualitative data analysis

Qualitative data were drawn out from the questionnaires using thematic analysis. Themes were identified from the two sample groups (i.e. health care workers and other professionals). The two groups were analysed separately at first and each case scrutinised individually, then comparisons between the groups and individual cases were made.

The sample

Of the original anticipated sample of 20 control (the non-HCW group) and 20 case (the HCW group), the final sample consisted of 12 HCWs and eight other professions ($n = 20$). It proved more difficult than anticipated to encourage people to come and discuss their experiences. Most people contacted were back at work and trying to piece their lives together again; they did not want to be reminded of their recent past experiences.

The HCW group consisted of six males and six females; the non-HCW group consisted of three males and five females. Ages of the participants ranged from 19 to 55 years of age (60 per cent in the 20–30 age range). There was no previous contact with the psychiatric services for nine of the 12 HCWs (75 per cent) and five out of the eight (62.5 per cent) non-HCWs. There was no family psychiatric history in ten HCWs (83 per cent) and five (62.5 per cent) non-HCWs.

The salary range varied from less than £4000 per annum to over £32,000 per annum for the HCWs, with the average salary falling between £13,000 and £14,000 per annum. For the non-HCW group the range was between £11,000 and £31,000, with the average salary falling between £17,000 and £19,000.

One HCW was employed on a part-time basis, whilst all other participants were in full-time employment. Both the HCW and non-HCW groups included four

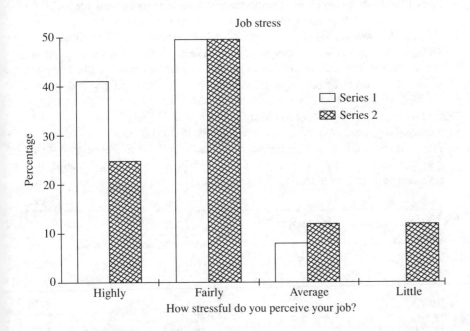

Figure 9.1 Series one represents the HCW group whilst series two represents the non-HCW group.

Table 9.1 Identified work stresses

Health care workers	Rank	Other professionals	Rank
Patients	1	Organizational bureaucracy	1
Time pressures and demands	2	Conflicting priorities/responsibility	2
Exams and study	3	Advocacy	3

people whose extra working hours ranged between 3 and 20 hours over and above their contractual expectation. Therefore 33 per cent of the HCW group and 66 per cent of the non-HCW group were working extra hours.

Forty-one per cent of the HCW group smoked but only 13 per cent of the non-HCW group did. Alcohol consumption was estimated by the groups in units per week and ranged from 0 to 21 units per week. Three HCWs denied drinking at all, whereas all non-HCWs admitted to drinking alcohol at levels between 1 and 15 units per week.

Job stress was identified using a five-point Lickert scale (Figure 9.1). In the HCW group, five people (41 per cent) rated their job as highly stressful (scored 1), six (50 per cent) rated it fairly stressful (a score of 2), and one person rated stress as average (score 3). In the non-HCW group, two people (25 per cent) rated their job highly stressful (1), four (50 per cent) fairly stressful (2), one person rated stress as average (3), and one other rated their job as a little stressful (4).

The two groups were asked to identify what they considered the most stressful part of their job. Using all the questionnaires, three categories were identified for each of the two groups and ranked in order of importance (Table 9.1).

Table 9.2 reveals the type of contact made by participants with a number of different agencies. The two sample groups were given the same list of possibilities and asked to indicate how many people they made contact with. The table shows the number of participants who responded. Interestingly both groups avoided contact with family members.

The HCWs' reasons for avoiding contact with helpers fell into two main themes. First the HCWs described a negative self-concept; this included feeling that their own patients were more depressed than themselves. The second theme was one of 'trust', for example not knowing where things would lead if they revealed how they were feeling (i.e. perhaps to disciplinary action) and also not

Table 9.2 Contacts made with agencies

Health care workers	Total	Other professionals	Total
Friend	2	Friend	7
Colleague	2	Colleague	1
Psychiatrist	1	Psychiatrist	2
Partner	2	Partner	4
Family	1	Family	0
Personal tutor	1	Community psychiatric nurse	1
General practitioner	2	General practitioner	2
Counsellor	0	Counsellor	3

having confidence in other professionals to help them. One participant said, 'My clients were more depressed than me'. Another person said, 'Hypothetically I hoped I'd just get better. I had very little insight into what was happening to me, events just overtook me.'

The interviewer asked whether sick leave or annual leave was taken as a means of coping. The non-HCW group took between zero and (for one participant) 246 days sick leave in one year. All eight participants recognized in retrospect that they were using annual leave as a coping strategy for the short-term effect it had on stress at work. Three of the group had fixed school holidays, which they recognized as something to look forward to which helped them to keep going. For the HCW group, sick leave ranged again from no time off at all up to 270 days in one year. Six people (50 per cent) stated they took around 20 sick days in the year, some in short blocks others in weeks at a time. The use of annual leave was more notably different for this group, for none said they took annual leave as a means of coping; one HCW admitted not having taken a holiday in four years. Most gave reasons for their absence to colleagues as due to a physical ailment (e.g. flu or back problems). 'If I'd have been anything but a doctor people would have said I needed time off'. The impression is that catastrophic events intervened as the HCW group struggled on at work until events simply took over. 'I was mugged and that was the last straw.' 'I collapsed at work,' another said. 'I'd been on a stress management course and the nurse came up to me afterwards and said she was worried about my depression. I was surprised; I didn't realize I was as depressed as I was.' 'I only turned to my GP when I wasn't coping on my course, they had suggested I take a year off, then I felt really bad.'

Finally we would like to present some of the comments made which concerned the participants' thoughts on what they would like to see change in care and treatment for occupational stress.

The non-HCW group

A *nursery nurse:* 'People have no idea what you are going through; it doesn't show and you can't have depression without a reason'. 'I wish I didn't feel it was a stigma but I'm right, you can't just ring up work and say, "I'm depressed, I can't come in today."'

A *personnel officer:* 'There needs to be some long or short term counselling available for people to help them deal with stress at work. I'm quite lucky as I work in a fairly open and caring environment; even so it's difficult to cope sometimes with all the pressures of the job. Mental health problems are still seen as a taboo or a sign of weakness.'

A *teacher:* 'Schools have become so insular. There was a child in our school killed by a train and there was nobody we could talk about it to professionally. There's no support network any more.'

A solicitor: 'There need to be more evening surgeries with marriage or career counsellors attached. I do hope there is more research into mental illness in our lifetime and that more information becomes available to us from the experts.'

A civil servant executive officer: 'There definitely needs to be more information available.'

A priest: 'I really don't know, as my awareness only came through a crisis.'

The HCW group

A student medic: 'People in general are reluctant to seek help about mental problems, more so in the medical profession – you're truly inhibited. In the role of a carer there are people at the other end who are not in such a powerful position as yourself, and, besides, who wants to be treated by the people you work with?'

A practice nurse: 'If things were more visible it wouldn't be so stigmatized. GPs should have something in their interviewing to pick up more on the emotional side of things, if someone had asked me it would have been a great release. I took on the physical ailments to get attention and some sympathy.'

A psychiatrist: 'I really didn't have any access to how I felt. I suppose on reflection I was worried about the embarrassment – what if the press got involved? There needs to be somewhere to go where people can be sensitive to your feelings and how to deal with them when you've been through the mill.'

A doctor: 'I thought I should be able to pull my socks up, I should know better. I think people who look after you as a fellow health worker think the same thing, and think you're just pathetic for not being able to cope as you should.'

An occupational therapist: 'In the health profession you think all the time: others first, yourself last. There need to be more counselling and advice services available, outside of the hospital you work in, or meeting up with other people who have similar problems.'

DISCUSSION

Much information has been obtained from this project despite the small sample size. It appears that most professional people have strong and fixed ideas as to how they should or should not behave. There is also a strong sense that suffering from a mental health problem is not as acceptable as physical problems and should remain unseen and unheard.

We did not anticipate the large proportion of people who were not willing to take part. Some were due to readmissions to psychiatric hospitals. One participant was on holiday in England and became unwell and then returned home to their native country. Others moved and could not be contacted. Two of the HCW sample are now deceased, one through a physical illness, the other a suicide. A large number did not wish to remember their breakdown and wished to put the past behind them. We aimed therefore to be particularly sensitive with the information being given and to deal carefully with the intrusive nature of the questions.

Guilt and inadequacy

Both groups of professionals discussed feelings of guilt about being unwell. The non-HCW group felt guilty about not coping and that they had to keep up a professional appearance – 'Other people saw me as a capable teacher' – whereas the HCWs' guilt lay in the need to care for others before caring for themselves, on top of the feeling they should be able to cope and know better.

Shame receives much less attention in psychiatry than anxiety, guilt, and depression. Freud (1896) interpreted shame as a fear of ridicule, whilst Piers and Singer (1953) interpreted it as a response to failure and trying to live up to one's ego ideal. In other words we feel shame if we fail to achieve an ideal we set ourselves. According to Lynd (1958) shame has a close connection with our sense of identity and insight. Shame is provoked by experiences that call into question our preconceptions about ourselves. It compels us to see ourselves through the eyes of others and to recognize the discrepancy of their perception of ourselves and our own oversimplified and egotistical conception of ourselves. If we face up to our feelings of shame, increased insight and self-awareness occur; if we deny it we become defensive (Rycroft, 1972).

Guilt differs from shame in that it relates to acts already committed. Guilty feelings are characterized by painful recollections of actions evaluated negatively and for which the person holds themselves responsible. Guilty feelings share with anger the idea that someone (the ego) is to blame as a causal agent: one could have acted otherwise; the situation could have been other than it is. Guilt feelings are often clung to in order to ward off a finality. Guilt gives rise to endless ruminations as to what could have happened had one acted otherwise (Frijda, 1986).

Reluctance to share

The HCWs' attitudes to sharing their experiences were polarized. Some were more than willing to participate in the project and felt they had changed their attitude to discussing more openly their experiences after the event whilst others were not willing to discuss any issue and even resented being contacted. One person contacted said, 'Can I not be allowed to forget the past?' It seems a pity when experiences cannot be shared in an attempt to encourage other people to learn and to help create a more needs-led service.

Secrecy

The secrecy expressed in nearly all the interviews was probably again to do with the strong feelings of guilt. Having to remain silent about their problems and not being able to share problems were recurrent themes for both professional groups. It will take a long time to find means of combating this secrecy. Helplines and counselling are available but little is known about them or what the consequences of seeking help might be. This sort of information availability needs urgent attention.

Professional identity

The HCW group expressed a recurrent theme of dealing with feelings of inadequacy as carers themselves. For professional carers, care was something to be lavished on others rather than something to be applied to themselves. Giving up, even for a short period, the role of carer and taking on that of being a patient is a difficult and exasperating experience. Most carers not only care at work but are invariably associated in that role within the home situation. It is a very hard task to give up one's identity, even for the sake of one's mental well-being.

It is significant therefore that health workers fail to seek help for themselves because of an overwhelming sense of guilt and shame associated with their professional actions and status.

CONCLUSIONS

The work of the health care workers' unit at the Bethlem and Maudsley has not been sufficient to save it as a specialist satellite unit. As with many projects this one leaves us with more questions than answers, but we hope it will give the reader some impression about the effect of caring for others on the mental health and well-being of the health profession. It is also important to recognize the strong connection of stress and identity experienced by the group of professionals. We can draw no clear-cut conclusions from the data presented here and would not wish to do so. It is perhaps pertinent to state again that one of the health care worker participants has subsequently taken her own life.

REFERENCES

Arnetz, B.B. (1991) White collar stress: what studies of physicians can teach us. *Psychotherapy and Psychosomatics*, **55** (2–4), 197–200.
Bailey, R.D. (1986) *Coping with Stress in Caring*, Blackwell Scientific Publications, Oxford.

Bale, R.N. (1986) The Sick Doctor. *British Medical Journal:* Update. 1022–8.

Beehr, T.A., Walsh, J.T. and Taber, T.D. (1976) Job role questionnaire. *Journal of Applied Psychology*, **61**, 41–7.

Brayfield, A.H. and Ruth, H.I. (1951) An index of job satisfaction. *Journal of Applied Psychology*, **35** (5), 307–11.

Caplan, R.P. (1994) Stress, anxiety and depression in hospital consultants, general practitioners and senior health service managers. *British Medical Journal*, **309**, 1261–3.

Cherry, N. (1978) Stress anxiety and work: a longitudinal study. *Journal of Occupational Psychology*, **51**, 259–70.

Cooper, C.L. and Kelly, M. (1993) Occupational stress in head teachers: a national UK study. *British Journal of Educational Psychology*, **63**, 130–43.

Dolan, N. (1987) The relationship between burnout and job satisfaction in nurses. *Journal of Advanced Nursing*, **12**, 2–12.

Freud, S. (1896) *Further Remarks on the Defence Neuro-psychosis*, 1962 edition. Vol. 3, Hogarth Press, London.

Frijda, N. H. (1986) *The Emotions: Studies in Emotion and Social Interaction*, Cambridge University Press, Cambridge.

Gibson (1966) Logical social inquiry. London.

House, R.J. and Rizzo, H.I. (1972) Anxiety stress questionnaire. *Organisational Behaviour and Human Performance*, **7**, 467–505.

Jackson, M. and Cawley, R.H. (1992) Psychodynamics and psychotherapy on an acute psychiatric ward. The story of an experimental unit. *British Journal of Psychiatry*, **160**, 41–50.

Jenkins, R. and Coney, N. (1992) In *Prevention of Mental Ill Health at Work*, HMSO, London.

Lynd, H.M. (1958) *On Shame and the Search for Identity*, Routledge and Kegan Paul, London.

Menzies-Lyth, E. I. (1989) *Containing Anxiety in Institutions. Selected essays*, vol. 1, Free Association Books, London.

Piers, G. and Singer, M. (1953) *Shame and Guilt*, C.C. Thomas, Springfield, IL.

Rycroft, C. (1972) *A Critical Dictionary of Psychoanalysis*, Penguin. London.

Tyler, P. and Cushway, D. (1992) Stress, coping and mental well being in hospital nurses. *Stress Medicine*, **8**, 91–8.

Waldegrave, W. (1991) In *Prevention of Mental Ill Health at Work*, HMSO. London.

Warr, P.B. and Payne, R.L. (1988) Experiences of strain and pleasure among British adults. *Social Science and Medicine*, **61**, 1691–7.

<table>
<tr><td>10</td><td># Providing support systems for health care staff</td></tr>
</table>

10 | Providing support systems for health care staff

Jan Long

Staff support in health care has become of increasing concern and interest. Organizations are looking at differing ways of helping staff who suffer the effects of caring. In fact it is now generally acknowledged that caring probably needs a 'government health warning'! 'Support' for health care workers has been highlighted with increasing frequency but what makes it so important?

There are four good reasons: (a) morality – no one can give what they do not receive; (b) quality in provision of services; (c) legality – health and safety legislation dictates the physical and mental care of staff; and, of course, (d) the costs. There are costs in human terms – of sickness, absenteeism, staff replacement, and medical retirement. In this chapter these costs will be examined in more detail alongside suggested strategies for managing the pressures of health care. The background to Swindon's staff support service is documented with case history supporting its use and effectiveness.

MORALITY

Health carers are, quite rightly, expected to be sensitive and compassionate to the needs of their patients and their families. Doctors often have to inform a patient that they will die, whilst nurses care for and comfort them, and then continue to support and care for bereaved relatives. Ambulance staff face fear, pain, and crisis as a daily part of their work. Midwives, health visitors, and GPs all deal with death in new-born babies and young children. These activities are not isolated incidents but occur as a regular part of the daily workload.

Sensitivity and compassion require immense emotional input from the professional carer yet they are often expected to ignore the impact of intense feelings on themselves in order to get the job done.

Staff are easily sucked into a self-destructive culture which demands that the 'patient comes first' whatever that may mean to the care giver. Jim George (1989) speaks of the lack of morality in health service culture. A culture that dictates that care staff deal compassionately with patients while ignoring the needs of those same staff is immoral. Whilst carers are taught to care compassionately, this is largely related to caring for patients and is not about caring for themselves or each other. He suggests that compassionate caring should not be limited to patients alone:

> if we believe in health (and if not why are we employed?), then we must believe in the health of our organisation and be committed to the health of our people – put another way it's about caring. ... If we care about our service then we must care about those who are dedicated to its ideals'.
> (George, 1989, p. 2)

QUALITY

There is a culture of vocation within the NHS and its training programmes. Over the years, public stereotypes of nurses as 'angels of mercy', altruistic and empathic, along with peer pressure to cope with the emotional labour of nursing, medicine, or management, have led carers to put themselves at the end of the queue for attention, leaving personal needs for care unmet.

NHS culture insists that 'if you cannot take the heat get out of the kitchen'. Workers think it is macho to start early and work late although quite clearly this is counterproductive in terms of time management, productivity, and quality service.

Of course the patient *is* crucially important, and so are the care staff, as Vaughan and Walsh (1986, p. 89) suggests: *'none can ask another to be healed but they can let themselves be healed and thus offer the other what he has received. Who can bestow upon another what he does not have? Who can share what he denies himself?'* If care staff feel disregarded, uncertain, isolated, vulnerable, or uncared for, then the service they provide for their patients will be profoundly and negatively affected.

Yet it also seems to be incredibly difficult for carers to face the challenge of admitting that they too have needs. While many staff are suffering the ill effects of stress at work, some are pretending these do not exist and others are still accepting the damage as 'normal' and to be expected in the field of health care. The majority are female; there has been a societal shift in family and household roles but there is still a great deal of evidence to suggest that the traditional role of women as carers in the community persists.

Many health care professionals will have role commitments related to caring outside their paid employment – as parents, spouses, or carers for family members. Role overload of this nature eventually takes its toll and women have been found to be vulnerable to 'burnout' and low job satisfaction because of role conflicts. (Anon, 1994)

THE PERSONAL COSTS OF CARING

Bailey (1986) defines the demands of caring as stressful and gives the following reasons:

- Caring may interfere with the health of the carer.
- Fear of admitting the need for help tends to exacerbate any existing distress.
- The burden of caring may progressively impair function to the point of burnout.

Cherness (1987) describes the process by which professional carers are affected by the stress of caring:

- The imbalance between the demands of the job and the personal resources of the individual.
- This leads to feelings of anxiety and exhaustion.
- Which in turn leads to a change in attitude and behaviour towards work, often characterized by emotional detachment, physical avoidance, apathy and cynicism.

Cherness (1987) comments that abuse of alcohol, drug taking, and physical symptomatology are frequent signals of distress. Cooper (1988) states that many nurses are now using negative coping strategies to survive the job. Plant *et al.* (1992) recorded that in 1986–1987 50 per cent of nurses reported to the UKCC Disciplinary Committee: their offences included drug and alcohol use. Negative forms of coping may have the adverse effect of leading to serious deficiencies in patient care delivery systems (Bailey 1986), which in turn can increase the distress of staff who truly wish to care compassionately for their patients. Health-damaging behaviours, emotional distress, and burnout may be the ultimate penalty for caring too much.

fiNANCIAL COSTS OF CARING

There is now substantial and growing evidence to support the increasing concerns for the physical and psychological health of professional care staff. Figures released from the Royal College of Nursing and the National Association for Staff Support (1992) record the financial costs: losing and replacing experienced nurses is costing the NHS up to £24 million every year. It costs £40,000–£50,000 to train and prepare a skilled, qualified nurse and another £3,000 each time a nurse leaves the NHS. Whilst not all nurses are leaving because of the stress in caring, anecdotal evidence from support services staff who work with 'distressed' carers indicate that these figures do include a significant number who find the job impacting too much on their physical, mental, or emotional health. Cutting the rate at which nurses leave the profession by only 15 per cent could save up to 6.4 million (Hancock, 1991). Stress in nurse training is also an enormous waste of resources. Birch (1975) recorded 66 per cent of a sample of nurses in the Newcastle area in

1969 as dropping out because they could not cope with the stress that nursing involved. The UKCC records show that these figures were replicated in 1986, identifying the attrition rate amongst learners as between 15 per cent and 30 per cent.

LEGALITY

The overview from the NHS management executive for 1996/1997 gives guidance on expectations of health care Trusts as good employers. The document makes particular reference to work-force planning, education and training, employment policy and practice, the development of team work, and staff welfare.

Health and safety legislation demands a 'duty of care' from the organization and makes particular reference to the importance of mental health as well as physical health and safety. The Walker versus Northumberland County Council case emphasizes the legal responsibility. John Walker was forced to take medical retirement from his senior social work post because of work-related stress. He won his case against his employer and received substantial damages. Costs to the organization are thought to have been more than £300,000.

The Ministry of Defence has recently also paid compensation to a Falklands veteran who suffered post-traumatic stress disorder as a result of poor debriefing. Other cases are currently being examined. It is suggested that employers face a surge of law suits from staff suffering stress.

POSITIVE OUTCOMES OF SUPPORTING STAFF

Research demonstrates that support systems not only help with job commitment and retention of staff but also have a direct effect on the quality of patient care. Dubovsky and colleagues (1977) reported on a support programme in a Coronary Care Unit. Where staff felt supported and listened to, they were identified as being more responsive to patients' needs. The study involved the regular completion of questionnaires at three-monthly intervals and the attendance at regular meetings to discuss the psychiatric aspects of patient care. Nurses were also asked to keep a log of direct patient contact each day.

Dubovsky and colleagues (1977) suggested that the improved support led to a reduction in staff anxiety levels, allowing them to be more alert to the minor but important changes in patients' condition, which led to increased feelings of security among patients. Earlier intervention appeared to reduce patient mortality and the increased security felt by patients shortened the length of stay in an expensive service facility, thus having a direct impact on service provision.

Vachon et al. (1978) highlighted similar findings when researching management of stress in a palliative care facility. On this occasion the focus was on management of the dying patient, their family, and staff reaction to patients with advanced cancer. Staff became aware that lack of understanding and acceptance of their own feelings had led to a lack of understanding of the feelings of their patients. Lack of trust among colleagues was created by personal perceptions of how they should be feeling as 'good nurses', instead of there being free expression of more normal grief reactions, such as anger, depression, frustration, helplessness, and hopelessness. Because of the lack of insight in themselves the nurses were unable to provide the emotional support necessary for patients and their families at this difficult time. Vachon (1978) clearly describes how this lack of insight led directly to a deterioration in patient care.

Through facilitated support groups these nurses were able to explore their own reactions. They began to accept their own emotional response as normal and were able to share with one another. They subsequently felt that they understood each other better and that similar emotions in patients were quite normal. They no longer had to force patients to repress or ignore feelings in order that the expected smooth interpersonal relationships should occur. Wilkinson (1991) confirms these findings in her research into nurses communicating with cancer patients. She described how 55 per cent of nurses interviewed from a specialist cancer hospital used blocking verbal behaviours which did not allow patients to express their emotions and fears. It seemed that amongst the factors that affected the staff response were the supportive nature of the environment on the ward and the attitude of the senior nurse in charge. If the charge nurse was a supportive and communicative role model, patient communication was facilitated.

THE SWINDON STAFF SUPPORT SERVICE

Towards the end of the last decade, the need for a support service in Swindon became more marked. There was not much statistical evidence, but the need was identified in a number of ways:

- The aftermath of the Hungerford shootings.
- Comments from the consultant psychiatrists that they were treating too many staff with work-related stress.
- Increasing concern from the Occupational Health Department that more and more absenteeism was stress related.
- Increasing pressure on staff from the NHS reforms.
- The increasing number of staff who for social or economic reasons were forced to work while coping with difficult domestic circumstances.
- The social stresses associated with living in one of the fastest growing towns in Europe, where the divorce rate is one of the highest in the country.

A clear need for support was established but the way of meeting it was less clear. At a superficial level, counselling could be provided, but even here there were difficulties to overcome; these are still a problem – though less so – six years later. Not all those in need have the skill or courage to recognize and deal with the problem themselves. Those who have sought help required immense reassurance about confidentiality and that they would not be branded a failure. Options to suit a range of different needs and prejudices needed to be found. It was important to find a solution that dealt not just with the effects of stress but also with the root causes. This meant changing the culture that traditionally exists within the NHS, particularly among nurses and doctors, whose training emphasizes the paramount needs of the patients but frequently fails to recognize the equally important needs of the carers.

WHAT IS STRESS?

This much used and abused term has gained the rather unfair reputation of being an imported American disease designed simply to provide employment for stress counsellors! In truth, stress is a perfectly normal reaction to a perceived threat – the fight or flight response to danger – and without a healthy stress response no human could have survived.

The stress response is vital for survival: it is the fight and flight escape mechanism. In health care, stress is necessary to react to emergencies, to cope with heavy demands, to be proactive, and to be healthy and enjoy life. Stress becomes 'distress' when pressures are unrelenting, when it is not always possible to rest, or when pressures come from several different directions at once. This leads to anxiety, frustration, disordered thinking, fear, and physical and mental health problems. Many problems for health carers tend to be a combination of home and work pressures. Where one is supportive, the other becomes manageable, but when both are troublesome the overload becomes a health risk.

It is, of course, totally unrealistic to expect health care workers to leave all their personal concerns at the door whilst at work, although this attitude is often expected. It is most frequently the combination of home worries and work pressure which creates the overload. The unhealthy and destructive working culture in health care leads staff to believe that to be seen not to cope is an admission of defeat and failure. This kind of environment creates cruelty and bullying and defies the belief that health carers actually care. If fear of failure drives the professional, then whose need is really being met – the patient's or the carer's?

WHO NEEDS SUPPORT?

The experience gained by the Swindon staff support team has shown that there are no groups of carers who do not need some form of support, whether employed in executive, administrative, clinical, or ancillary work. Pressure is placed on managers to comply with major reforms. Their subordinates struggle to implement decisions with insufficient resources. Junior staff learn in unfamiliar areas. Workers face personal demands such as financial pressures, health worries, family sickness, or bereavement.

PRINCIPLES UNDERLYING THE PREFERRED SOLUTION

Once it was acknowledged that a support system would be of value, and following many discussions, the following principles were identified as vital if the eventual solution was to prove successful. These principles established in 1988 remain as valuable today as they were then.

- The service must be recognized, supported, and promoted at the very top of the organization, so that it will be accepted as part of the new culture.
- The service must deal not just with counselling but with those features of life which lead to stress.
- The service must not undermine the authority of managers.
- Confidentiality must be guaranteed.
- All aspects of the service, but especially the counselling, must be provided on a professional basis.
- The service must set a good example by ensuring that those who provide it are well supported themselves.
- To satisfy financial restrictions and the need to involve key managers the service should have at its core those already in the organization who have the skills, understanding, and experience to deliver the service.

SWINDON STAFF SUPPORT SERVICE STRATEGY

The unique strategy adopted by the Swindon Staff Support Centre attempts to meet these principles by encouraging a variety of initiatives throughout the organization. It attempts, through personal development training – with groups or individuals, using mind and body work – to encourage and empower staff to find their own healthy coping strategies. This means that issues likely to lead to excess stress can be defused long before they cause disruption through illness or absenteeism. It also encourages the use of skilled practitioners already within the Trusts to use their skills to support colleagues from other similar organizations. This reciprocal arrangement has the advantage of valuing staff who are already employed. Costing only their time and supervision, the service encourages the compassionate culture to develop. This has the additional benefit of affecting patient care standards as previously described.

IMPLEMENTING THE SERVICE

In November 1989 a questionnaire was circulated. The aims of the survey were:

- To discover the extent of awareness, understanding, and need for support strategies.

- To highlight the main areas of concern for staff.
- To determine what interventions would be of most value.

As a result of this and the subsequent acceptance of a 'case of need' by the previous District Health Authority, a support services coordinator was appointed, initially on a part-time basis. The resulting demand very quickly highlighted the need for the post to be full-time. Since then the service has gradually grown and developed, and found its base in the new Trusts structure, providing a broad range of support strategies through NHS Trusts and other caring agencies. There is also interest from non-NHS businesses who have seen the value of staff care and are looking at the current model provided for health carers as an example of good practice.

The service helps to address the mental, physical, and emotional needs of health care workers across the district. It began with some small-scale communication skills workshops and personal counselling for staff who were self-referred. Over the last six years, however, the service has grown to a fully functioning multidisciplinary team of 14 members working together to promote the mental and physical health of professional carers. The team currently consists of seconded volunteers, physical therapists, trainers, and sessionally paid counsellors, as well as psychotherapists working within the Code of Ethics of the British Association of Counselling or the United Kingdom Council for Psychotherapy.

The service has also been approved as a placement for postgraduates studying for an MA in counselling who need professionally supervised clinical practice. The service has attracted a high calibre of senior students who are already professionally qualified and are seeking further qualifications. The service philosophy dictates that health care workers should not join a long waiting list for psychological care: this combination of staff provides a professional yet cost-effective service, enabling carers to be seen well within the standard target of two weeks.

Strategies for staff support include the recognition and prevention as well as the treatment of stress-related problems. A variety of support programmes are in place aimed at maintaining the mental and physical health of the individual worker, rather than patching people up and sending them back to the front line as walking wounded. However, the first-aid measures designed to deal with work-damaged staff remain a vital if frustrating aspect of the service.

CENTRAL FEATURES OF THE CURRENT SERVICE

Personal development training

Training includes counselling skills, breaking bad news, handling verbal aggression and bullying, and dealing with loss, grief, and bereavement. The service also provides workshops in time management, assertiveness, relaxation, and meditation. Through training and personal development, staff are encouraged to ask for or provide the changes necessary to manage the pressures of health care themselves.

Counselling and psychotherapy

The service has an increasing number of counsellors and psychotherapists working both within and independently of the NHS. They offer a wide variety of approaches, which allows clients a choice. All carry full indemnity insurance and follow the Code of Ethics of the British Association for Counselling or the United Kingdom Council for Psychotherapy. All attend regular professional supervision.

In April 1995 the service was given its own dedicated base – the Staff Support Centre. The number of clients has gradually increased over the years. With the launch of the new centre in April 1995 the numbers have more than doubled. Much of the increased use is due to the increased publicity since the opening of the centre. Those who access one aspect of the service often return to use another. For example, staff attending a training workshop will meet some of the team and feel safe enough to return for professional support or counselling.

Professional support (group and individual)

It is only natural that senior staff, both clinical and managerial, find problems associated with their role; it is not always appropriate to discuss them with subordinates or line managers, particularly if those same managers are responsible for assessment or individual performance review. The professional support sessions allow managers and isolated professionals to access a confidential space in which to examine a work-related or personal difficulty. These sessions tend to be less regular than counselling appointments but since their inception in late 1994 have become increasingly popular. They are seen not as an emotional crutch but rather as a constructive personal and professional development activity.

Meditation and relaxation groups

It has been emphasized throughout that many stressful situations should be addressed at an organizational level. However, it is essential to offer personal strategies to complement organizational change. Workshops to encourage the individuals to value themselves are a fundamental necessity because health care staff find it so hard to do so.

PERSONAL STRESS CARE PROGRAMMES

A small number of staff who were on long-term sick leave with stress-related problems were offered a combined, personally tailored programme of care using the range of services available. These staff had manifested stress through physical problems such as high blood pressure, migraine, back pain, chest pain, and digestive disorders.

An initial assessment by the staff support service was followed by an intensive, negotiated programme based on an holistic mind, body, and spirit approach. Each programme contained a counselling/psychotherapy component, a body therapy such as aromatherapy massage, reflexology or shiatsu, and yoga, meditation, or a relaxation programme to be practised at home. In all cases the presenting physical problems continued to be monitored by the person's own GP. All reported substantial improvements in their physical symptoms within the first week of their programme. They also reported qualitative, measurable general health improvements. All were able to return to work earlier than anticipated. Some requested and received ongoing support after their return to work. This is provided during the working day – which emphasizes the commitment of both staff and managers to the work of the service.

Complementary therapies

Subsidised aromatherapy, yoga, shiatsu, and reflexology are available both independently and through the personal stress care programmes; one Trust has even increased the subsidy through its staff lottery in order to help the less well paid to access these services. This is an example of a good staff care philosophy which costs the organization nothing yet enhances goodwill enormously.

TYPES OF DISTRESS ENCOUNTERED BY THE STAFF SUPPORT SERVICE

Since its inception the staff support service has identified seven types of stress affecting health care workers in the district.

Positive pressure

This is vital for managing everyday work pressures and emergencies but is often required so continuously and to such a degree that overload occurs and tiredness renders the positive element ineffective for quality working practice.

CASE HISTORY

A ward manager began to be concerned that his memory was no longer as effective and he was becoming increasingly irritable at home and work. He was also aware that he was avoiding colleagues and staff meetings. He saw increasing minor sickness amongst his staff and a general low morale. Team members, normally cheerful and helpful to each other, were short tempered and uncooperative. He was concerned enough to ask for some individual professional support in order to try to understand what was happening. Through this system he was able to look at the effect of the NHS changes on individual staff and began to recognize both his own and his team's anxieties. He realized that they were all trying to introduce the reforms and keep up good standards of practice on top of all their pre-existing roles. He introduced ward 'away days' and support meetings in service time, asked the staff support service to facilitate team-building workshops, and enabled his team to air their concerns. The impact of these non-clinical activities enabled the whole team to support each other and energized them to discover creative ways to manage the work pressure. Although the pressure continues, the team response has reduced the unhealthy effects on individuals and provided a cohesive team approach to problem solving.

Quantitative work overload

This is often found in senior clinical and managerial staff. There is too much to do, with too little time in which to do it. Staff work longer and longer hours in the effort to be seen as coping with their work overload. Irritation, frustration, avoiding contact with subordinates and their problems, and work avoidance through absenteeism and sickness are some of the observed outcomes of overload. Anxiety about job safety has created a newer condition called presenteeism. The employee is present but not functioning to their normal capacity, afraid to take sick leave for fear of losing their job.

CASE HISTORY

A senior manager responsible for a larger department gradually found herself less able to concentrate, making mistakes and feeling generally unwell. She could not understand this since she was a steady, very hard working manager who had never had any problems over the many years she had worked for the NHS. Over the last months her workload had increased as colleagues left and were not replaced and on some occasions she worked until 10.00 p.m. and returned to her office at 6.00 a.m.

Initially, she felt unable to discuss this with her manager as she thought she might be the next to go. With the firm encouragement and support of her GP she reluctantly took time out and then, with considerable courage, accessed the staff support service to look at the issues. It did not take her long to realize the extent to which work had become her life, to the exclusion of her family and the detriment of her mental and physical health. After some weeks' realignment of life priorities and reassessment of her work schedule she is well and back at work – for office hours only!

Cumulative stress or compassion overload

This is commonly found in staff from specialist clinical units such as hospices or care of the dying, accident and emergency departments, and other intensive-care working environments. Staff can become immersed in and eventually over-whelmed by the emotions associated with sudden or lingering death, although they have often been unaware of their deep involvement until sickness has intervened.

CASE HISTORY

A single career nurse, having spent many years in different posts, finally set-tled for nursing the terminally ill. She was and still is a very compassionate and caring professional. Over a period of many months she began to realize that she was no longer enjoying the work and actively avoiding patient con-tact whenever she could. She became susceptible to frequent minor illnesses and began taking time off sick. Fortunately her experienced and compas-sionate manager knew her well and, rather than using disciplinary proce-dures, suggested accessing staff support. Using a combination of psychological support and body therapies this nurse was able to recognize that in her need to be effective as a carer she had denied her own needs to be cared for. She was physically and emotionally exhausted from giving. From an intensive start to a continual programme of regular aromatherapy and pro-fessional support this nurse is back on form, working well and very aware of her own needs and those of her subordinates.

Post-traumatic stress

A normal reaction to an abnormal event. However, where such events are being experienced on top of a professional health-care role, the stress can be over-whelming. Events that staff have brought to the attention of the service include, for example, physical assault, rape, witnessing a suicide, and involvement in a fatal road accident in which a child was killed.

CASE HISTORY

A young nurse working on an acute ward was on night duty when a new patient admitted earlier in the day for investigations asked if he could smoke. The nurse escorted him to the appropriate room where he noticed the patient's agitation. Having reported this to his team leader, he was returning to collect the patient and became aware of the cold draught of an open win-dow as he neared the room. On entering he was in time to see his patient fall from the open window to his death.

The nurse was a competent and compassionate general nurse, unused to mentally ill clients and was profoundly affected by the memory of this ter-rible incident. This abnormal experience would for any nurse cause a post-traumatic stress reaction. He was unable to sleep, suffering flashbacks and nightmares. He also felt his confidence ebbing, fearing a repeat episode and was unable to return to the ward. With his ward manager's support he and his colleagues attended the staff support service for a formal psychological debrief. He returned for follow-up, receiving a total of four and one half hours input from the service. Within 14 days he was back at work and functioning normally.

Personal life crisis

Bereavement, divorce, or financial problems, in addition to a professional caring role, may be too much to bear, again producing overload.

CASE HISTORY

A mature married carer working voluntarily with the mentally ill was asked to co-facilitate a group for sexual abuse survivors. This went well for some months until she began to realize that she was re-experiencing her own painful memories which she had until this time forgotten. About this time the abuser, a close family member, suddenly died. This, with her awakening memories, led to a deterioration in her relationship with her partner and the potential for their marriage to break up. She sensibly asked for some personal help and professional support in order to separate the issues. She continues to work on her own experiences in therapy and has been able to share these with her partner, who has proved to be immensely supportive. She has been able to continue working with the mentally ill in another capacity.

Bullying and harassment at work

The current levels of anxiety and fear brought on by the major cultural change within health care have led to an undercurrent of 'personal survival strategies'. Among the techniques developed, frequent low-grade bullying often goes unnoticed; if challenged, staff are shocked to realize that this is actually happening. A growing number of staff using the service raised issues of bullying and several were eventually forced to take medical retirement on the grounds of mental ill health.

Lyons, Tivey and Ball (1995) list a summary of current bullying behaviours:

- Shouting and abusing, undermining confidence.
- Humiliation and ridicule.
- Excessive supervision and criticism about minor things.
- Taking credit but never accepting blame and overruling authority.

Bullying can also take the following forms:

- Reducing areas of responsibility.
- Setting impossible objectives or constantly changing the work remit.

- Withholding information.
- Ostracizing and marginalizing the victim.
- Spreading malicious rumours.
- Refusing requests for leave and training.

It is often difficult to differentiate between firm management and bullying but these guidelines may make it easier for staff and managers alike.

CASE HISTORY

A group of senior managers were discussing tactics for getting staff to conform to the changes and cost savings currently necessary. When the subject of bullying was raised, all were profoundly shocked to discover that this was exactly what they were doing.

Combinations of causes of stress

Combinations of the above can result in major distress, physical and mental health breakdown, and burnout.

CASE HISTORY

An experienced and well respected manager suffered two close family bereavements and her partner's redundancy at a time of major change at work. Redundancies in her own department were possible and both she and her colleagues were very anxious. Personal finances became a worry, mixed with her natural grief. She became anxious and insecure; her work began to suffer. Her anxiety led to sleepless nights, poor health, disrupted eating patterns and increased alcohol consumption. There was further deterioration in her personal relationships and standards of work which finally led to a warning for poor performance.

She took a personal decision to access individual counselling, in which she was able to address in confidence her personal feelings of lack of control. Later, with her doctor's support, she took time out to recover her health using a support service combined mind and body programme. Having gained insight into her behaviour, she was able to meet with her line manager to explain the situation. Once he understood the situation clearly she received clear guidance and support from him and a planned return to work enabled her to reclaim her previous standards of work.

Organizational stress

An increasingly important aspect of the work in Swindon is that of addressing organizational solutions rather than directing efforts towards individuals only. Personal interventions such as counselling, while useful, can sometimes be seen at best as patching up the wounded before returning them to the battlefield. It is clear that a major increase in service use has been noticed throughout the period of the change to Trust status. Fear is the most commonly presented sign of organization dysfunction and it has a capacity to spread rapidly throughout the service, affecting individual health and operational efficiency as described earlier in this chapter.

It is also important to emphasize that, whilst concerned support and counselling at work may be a useful tool, in legal terms it should not be seen as the final solution to organizational pressures on staff. Dr Michael Carol, Lecturer in Psychology at the Roehamton Institute, suggests that in-house counselling alone may be insufficient to protect employers from claims. He advised at a recent seminar that unless organizations were prepared to look at their internal culture and reduce excessive demand, then counselling alone would be seen as an attempt to shift the blame from the Trust to the individual.

Reports and statistics

The service provides regular reports and statistical breakdown to the Trust managers, showing increases in use, trends, and concerns expressed. This is done using non-attributable data collection. There is, however, a danger of 'shooting the messenger' in the case of reports that are not nice reading for executives. Support services providers should be aware of the potential for compromise when your salary depends on the Trust managers and more importantly on maintaining the trust and confidence of staff while fulfilling an ethical responsibility to feed back professionally to Trust leaders. It is vital for the service to be seen to be separate from, and independent of, both management and staff-side organizations.

EVALUATION

The Swindon staff support system has been shown to be effective in both individual stress reduction and the impact this can have at the organizational level. The 'Health of the Nation Targets for Health for All 2000' (Department of Health, 1991) provides an impetus to all organizations, as well an obligation within the NHS, as the major supplier of health, to broaden the support remit and to be an exemplar of positive mental and physical health programmes.

Effective staff support means creating a culture that cares at least as much about its employees as it does about its users. For many years the NHS has survived on the goodwill and overworking of its staff. That goodwill is now running out. Staff are slowly beginning to accept their own need for compassionate care in order to give compassionate care to patients. Compassion should be good management employment practice for staff as well as patients. As George (1989, p. 4) states, 'to be fully effective carers need to feel cared for ... at the most basic level they need to be empowered and encouraged to care for themselves'.

The Health Authority for Wiltshire and Bath, East Wiltshire Health Care NHS Trust, and other Swindon Trusts and charities have now recognized this – in the establishment and continued backing of the staff support service. The service is acknowledged to have had a positive impact on the mental and physical health of the large number of staff who have used it over the years since it began, and specifically through its integrated programme approach. Services are now provided to a broad group of health care workers from the voluntary sector, primary care, hospitals, and community settings; increasingly, non-NHS organizations are asking for services. When non-health-care industrial managers see that supporting their own staff makes for good profits, it is time health carers' needs were taken very seriously indeed. The staff support service also leads the phase two psychological response to a major incident in North Wiltshire by liaising with local agencies likely to be involved, such as social services, police, local church ministers, and the voluntary sector. This work complements the debriefing already provided to health care workers, by training a wider community group to reach others likely to be involved.

The service cannot solve every problem. There are many intractable issues, like the organization that denies it has a problem despite the obvious evidence of distress; or when a member of staff is medically retired due to a work-induced stress-related illness, despite our best endeavours. It can be hard to believe that cultural change will ever happen. But then we remember those who have found the service useful. Frequent comments from support service users make us feel better and remind us of the importance of caring about those who give, as well as those who receive what is willingly offered:

- 'Thank you for being there; I know that I would have done something foolish if you weren't.'
- 'Thank you for being there when I needed you; you will never know how much you kept me on the straight and narrow!'
- The manager who evaluated a short-term team-building group said that 'it was so valuable that it was cost effective to continue it on a long-term basis'.
- A report from a service manager who expressed an opinion that 'the staff support service had kept me at work'.
- Evaluation on a training event: 'To me it was more than just a course; its effects and the learning will stay with me for ever.'

While this service has been recognized as one of the leaders in the field by both the Institute of Personnel Managers and the Royal College of Nursing, this is not enough. The cost-effective benefits to the service have only begun to be demonstrated. It is time for all health care staff to consider support mechanisms as important a part of their employment practice as paid annual leave and to actively develop appropriate systems to suit their own needs.

The National Association for Staff Support (NASS) is supporting local services through advice and help to members, its programme of conferences, and its collection of reference papers on all aspects of support. NASS creates a network of those interested in the field of staff support, allowing a sharing of skills and ideas. Its members come from a wide range of disciplines – from nurses and psychiatrists to chaplains, occupational health physicians, counsellors, psychotherapists, and personnel managers. The need now is to provide the empirical evidence to demonstrate this in a wider arena. NASS members are currently beginning this important work.

NASS can be contacted at: 9 Caradon Close, Woking, GU21 3DU; telephone 01483 771599.

REFERENCES

Anon (1994) Burnished or burnt out: the delights and dangers of working in health. *Lancet*, **344**, 8937.

Bailey, R.D. (1986) *Coping with Stress in Caring*, Blackwell Scientific Publications, Oxford.

Birch, J. (1975) *To Nurse or Not to Nurse*, Royal College of Nursing.

Cooper, C. (1988) *Living with Stress*, Penguin, Harmondsworth.

Cherness, C. (1987) *Staff Burnout – Job Stress in the Human Services*, Sage Publications, London.

Department of Health (1991) *Health of the Nation: a Consultative Document for Health*. HMSO, London.

Dubovsky, S.L., Getto, C.J., Adams Gross, S. and Paley, J.A. (1977) Impact on nursing care and mortality: psychiatrists on a coronary care unit. *Psychosomatics*, August, 18–27.

Fowler, F.G. and Fowler, H.W. (1992) *Oxford English Dictionary*, Clarendon Press, Oxford.

George, J. (1989) *Stressed Staff – Why Should Managers be Concerned?* King's Fund Centre.

Hancock, C. (1991) *Nursing Standard*, **6**, 3.

Lyons, R,. Tivey, H. and Ball C. (1995) *Bullying at Work and How to Tackle It*, MSF Health and Safety Office, London.

Nursing Standard (1991) A caring profession? **5**, 46.

Plant, M., Plant, M. and Foster, J. (1992) Stress, Alcohol, tobacco and illicit drug use amongst nurses: a Scottish study. *Journal of Advanced Nursing*, **17**, 1057–67.

RCN (1992) *Costs of Stress and the Cost Benefits of Stress Management.* The National Association for Staff Support, by The Royal College of Nursing, London.

Ross, C.E. and Mirowsky, J. (1988) Child Care and Emotional Adjustment to Wives Employment. *Journal of Health and Social Behaviour*, **29**, 127–38.

Tabnor, A.R. (1989) *Nursing Care: Theory and Practice*, Churchill-Livingstone, Edinburgh.

Vachon, M.L., Lyall, W. and Freeman, S. (1978) Measurement and management of stress in health professionals working with patients with advanced cancer. *Death Education*, **1**, 365–74.

Vaughan, F. and Walsh, R. (1986) *A Gift of Peace*, St Martins Press, New York.

Wilkinson, S. (1991) Communicating with Cancer Patients. *Nursing Standard*, **5**, 54.

The staff support group as a monitor for work-related stress: a personal perspective

11

Mark Sutherland

The phone rings and the voice on the other end identifies herself. My memory is jogged and I recall that she was at one time a member of a staff support group I facilitated before she moved to her present position on another unit. She asks me if I would consider facilitating a similar group on her current unit. A mixture of feelings flow through my mind – 'I have no time' – 'With five groups, already no vacancy' – 'What do they really want'? – 'Isn't this good, another unit asking for a group' – 'It's flattering to be asked' – 'There is such a lot of need out there; how can I refuse?' But the fact is I have no vacancy for another group and I suggest she approach the staff counsellor, the psychotherapy department, and then finally suggest I will speak to one of my part-time chaplain colleagues. I put the phone down and begin to think about how to convince Barry, my colleague, to offer this unit at the very least an exploratory consultation.

Staff support groups are part of the unofficial culture of my institution, a psychiatric hospital. Unofficial because they are hardly ever formally recognized by reference to the other indicators that identify work activity. For instance, there is usually no budget for them, hence a facilitator has to be found from within the institution who will do it for nothing. Attendance is 'voluntary' and does not usually include the most powerful and influential members of the multidisciplinary team. In short, some think it is a good idea, some don't, but it is not really part of the 'work'. After all it is only 'support'!

I am filled with wonder at how the subculture of such groups continues to survive as a kind of protest (particularly from sections of the staff who feel most put upon) against a more aggressive caricature of the official 'work-oriented' culture of the institution. However, herein lie the miracle and the dilemma, the prospect for hope and the reason to despair. I believe that staff support groups are potentially powerful instruments for registering the stress of the work and the institutional setting for the work. However, it is the messenger not the message which is found to be at fault. An instrument that registers distress is easily mistaken for the source of the distress.

The medium of the group has two advantages over more individualistic foci upon stress. The nature of most work is collaborative. We know from personal experience that collaboration is difficult and at times emotionally costly. Through action research based studies we have known for a long time that the way we organize the performance of the work has little to do with ensuring task efficiency (Menzies Lyth, 1988, 1989). Despite the collaborative, collective nature of most work, we continue to emphasize the individual within the work. Contemporary emphasis on individual performance is intensified by approaches to stress management which perceive the ability or failure to manage stress as an individual problem. But if work is collaborative then some aspects of task performance and resulting stress become visible only when viewed through the collective instrument of a group. Only a group is able to reveal the unconscious collective processes, the management of which contributes to, or diverts from, collaborative task performance. Individuals taken severally can be seen to have a role to play in the registration of stress, but to look only at individuals is to exacerbate the processes fragmenting the whole picture. The group forms a concrete matrix where processes hidden by their fragmentation and dispersal across the face of an institution and its work take form and become observable.

> A unit over some years had developed an infamous reputation for being a lethal place for nurses to work. Despite the constant turnover of staff, somehow a culture of persecution was passed on down the generations of those who worked there. At one point a serious breakdown in relations between the nursing manager and the primary nurses occurred. The nurses wrote a letter of complaint about their manager, and eventually achieved her removal to another unit. This simply reinforced the wider view of this unit held generally in the hospital. Over a period of time as facilitator to the unit's staff support group, I made interpretations designed to link what had gone on between the nurses to the work and the institutional environment. These interpretations had a limited effect. The members of the group found them interesting, but seemed unable to trust that greater understanding could lead to change.

This unit formed an intersection between a number of unconscious dynamic processes that characterized the institution as a whole. This was why the unit performed such a successful scapegoat role as evidenced by the significance of its reputation. In the group the following institutional processes became observable:

(1) This unit was an amalgamation of two different specialities which did not fit well together. This was dealt with in the usual way by a complete communi-

cation split between the two medical teams. However, the nurses nursed both groups of patients and bridged the medical divide. The latent tensions between medical specialities came together as conflict within the nursing group.

(2) Within an institution like a hospital there is always to be found a tension between clinical and managerial priorities. The tension is managed by negotiation between separate persons or groups representing these priorities. However, the recent philosophy of devolving managerial responsibility downwards has resulted in the senior nurse being turned from a clinical leader into a manager. Here this resulted in the tension between the clinical and the managerial being lodged in one group, i.e. nursing, where it became played out as conflict within the nursing group. The process of devolving responsibility also serves the function of merging, and thus obscuring, lines of conflict.

In both (1) and (2) conflict that belonged more generally within the institution became projected and concretized in one group within one unit. The conflict was not necessarily unique to this unit, but the process was magnified by the following:

(3) A dynamic characteristic of one of the medical conditions the unit treated was a state of persecutory confusion between the patients and their families. Was it something in the family system that persecuted the patient, resulting in the patient's illness? Or was it the patient resorting to illness to persecute the family? This became reflected in the behaviour between nurses: everyone felt persecuted, which led them to perpetrate acts of persecution.

'SUPPORT' – A PROBLEMATIC CONCEPT

Words are never neutral, in the sense that they can be seen as mere descriptors. Words occur within systems of meaning encoded with particular connotations. The hospital is such a system of meaning and within its work culture the word 'support' takes on different meanings across divergent professional cultures. Interactions and interrelations between the professional identities of nursing, medicine, and management create the institutional work culture which permeates each and every support group. The culture created by these interrelations produces an environment where the negotiation of conflict forms the basis for cooperation and an enhancement of a work culture. However, when interrelations are characterized by high levels of anxiety concerning competition and difference an environment is created where processes of splitting and collusion replace open negotiation of conflict.

Within the institutional work culture of the psychiatric hospital, I have noticed the way 'support' is often encoded with the connotation of 'weakness'. Needing 'support' is tantamount to an admission of not being able to cope.

Being able to cope is defined by professional attitudes to the work task. Medical, nursing, and management cultures each have highly 'instrumental' attitudes towards the work task. The work is to 'do' to the patient, who endures having things 'done' to them by the professional carers. This leads to the stereotype that the carers have to cope or cannot admit to not coping, because to not cope is to be closely identified with the state of being a patient. In the psychiatric institution this is a dangerous identification.

Menzies Lyth (1988) has demonstrated how and why the identification by carer with patient is unavoidable. For an extensive exploration of the mechanism of projection and identification between career and patients, see Menzies Lyth's discussion of this in her paper 'The functioning of social systems as a defense against anxiety' in Menzies Lyth (1988). This helps us to understand why 'support' provokes so much anxiety. I referred to the image of carers as copers and patients as those needing support as a stereotype because, like most stereotypes, while containing some truth, it acts to obscure matters that are a good deal more complex than this. An exploration of the interrelationship between professional groups within the wider work culture further reveals that while it is often difficult for doctors and managers to admit to needing support, nurses continually complain about their need for, and lack of, support.

Each professional group occupies a slightly different position within the work culture in relation to the patients. I would characterize this difference in position as one of distance from the recipients of care. Needing to be cared for is one of the sources of unconscious anxiety arising within the work of the caring institution. Put crudely, managers manage the structures, doctors manage the treatment, while nurses support the patient. This brings nurses into much closer physical and emotional proximity to the stigmatized patient culture. This proximity leaves nurses more exposed to the interface between caring and being cared for. It is along this interface that 'support' becomes identified with weakness and human frailty (Menzies Lyth, 1988). Here 'support' equates with feeling vulnerable.

If nurses are in closer proximity to the anxiety generated by being a patient, the doctors and managers, protected from this anxiety by an increased distance from the patient, nevertheless experience anxiety resulting from higher levels of accountability. Our society believes in science and regulates itself through political structures of a highly administrative nature. These two areas, one concerning knowledge, the other concerning power, each form a different interface along which doctors and managers find themselves likewise exposed to powerful unconscious anxieties. Both science and politics are not easily permeable to identifications with human weakness and frailty. This helps to explain why 'support' for these professional groups takes on a pejorative connotation. Here 'support' equates with being incompetent.

'THE GROUP' – ANOTHER PROBLEMATIC CONCEPT

The very mention of the word 'group' evokes powerful responses. 'I hate groups'; 'groups are cruel'; 'people do things in groups they wouldn't dream of doing by themselves'; 'I wouldn't want to join any group that would have me as a member'.

In health-care circles the natural human anxieties associated with group membership have been compounded by two other factors. The first is the legacy of the 1960s fashion for encounter and T groups. These have left a stereotype of groups as self-indulgent, left wing, emotionally disinhibited, old fashioned, and an inefficient waste of time. Secondly the association of groups with group therapy has left many believing that membership of a 'group' is a sign that things are not quite right with you. Yet, most of us participate in groups quite a lot of the time. We often disguise this fact by calling them meetings and rigidly constructing them around very clear agenda and statements of purpose and objective. Meeting in groups is a necessary prerequisite for work to take place. A difficulty arises when the process guiding the execution of the task becomes subverted by activity aimed at defending the workers against undue levels of stress. Defence becomes an unacknowledged substitute for work. The current obsession with documenting work is a good example here.

Bion (1987) identified two different aspects to a group's experience. He termed these 'work group' and 'basic assumption group' activity. Work group activity is where the individual members of a group maintain strong individual identities while at the same time joining in a collaborative venture. The key to this is the way the work group manages the elements of difference and conflict between members. The work group possesses a capacity for learning based on the negotiation of difference in experience of its members. It unitizes the different perspectives and experiences of its members in a developmental manner. Verbal communication in the work group allows for collaborative thinking because it remains possible for individual members to hold and think their own thoughts.

Basic assumption activity takes over from work group activity when the levels of unconscious anxiety concerning differences (i.e. anxieties about cooperation versus competition, fear of loss of identity versus collaborative individuality) between members rise to the point where the purpose of activity switches from managing the task to managing the anxiety within the group. Because this is unconscious the switch is not apparent to the members of the group. When this occurs developmental learning stops, as thinking is replaced by reactive fantasies and unexamined assumptions which come to be powerfully and collusively shared between group members. Here conflict comes to be feared. Conflict arising from natural differences between members has become a feared difference between each individual member and the group. For each member to challenge as a way of asserting his or her own thoughts is to fall foul of the rest of the group. Collusion replaces creative conflict. Verbal communication becomes empty talking, chatter-filled intermissions in an overwhelming atmosphere of stuck silence.

A particular group had begun to respond over a period of time to a supportive and open style of leadership from its consultant. The staff support group was used as a forum for examining the internal dynamics of the team as it struggled with a very difficult type of work in a hostile and punishing administrative environment. The functioning of the group suddenly changed when the consultant unexpectedly announced he was leaving. Communication between members over succeeding weeks was replaced by futile chatter punctuating paralysed silence. Each person seemed to be retreating into isolation. I interpreted that what members now shared was this increasing feeling of isolation from one another, the result of a crisis in the leadership of the team. An atmosphere of keeping one's head down (flight) developed. The discussion that took place was always about how hostile the outside world was and how pointless it was to register any kind of protest. I took this to be an indirect communication about the nature of the anxiety within the team. Anger towards the consultant could not be consciously expressed in the group. The need to express anger was replaced by a feared fantasy of anger. This made the atmosphere in the team feel potentially destructive and frightening. The group adopted basic assumption flight in the face of the unconscious anger now poisoning relations between members.

All professional cultures employ groups to facilitate the work task. Whether these are called a debriefing group, ward round, clinical review, or business meeting makes little difference to the behaviour of people within the collective setting. All groups contain both work group and basic assumption group characteristics. Both types of behaviour relate to all group situations, applying to different phases of the group's negotiation of its work task. I have sat in committees where the basic assumption behaviour, i.e. behaviour designed for defensive management of unconscious anxiety rather than collaborative task achievement, has been every bit as powerful as anything I have encountered in experiential group settings. All groups will switch back and forth between work group and basic assumption group behaviour. Menzies Lyth has commented on the importance to the health of our institutions of understanding both unconscious and conscious levels of functioning. She comments:

> Of particular significance are the defences developed to deal with anxiety-provoking content and difficulties in collaborating to accomplish the common task. These defences appear in the structure of the institution itself and permeate its whole way of functioning. (1989, p. 28)

Within my institution a curious distinction is made between staff support groups and all other types of group activities. One recognizes a rhetoric of disparagement: 'indulgent', 'waste of time', and 'navel gazing' are some of the ways the staff support groups are critically characterized. I am the first to admit that they can and often are deserving of all these criticisms, but why are the criticisms only applied to staff support groups and not to management committees and strategy planning groups, medical ward rounds and research reviews? I suggest the answer lies in the way these descriptions of group activity avoid reference to the words 'group' or 'support'. Anxiety raised by the mere mention of either of these words indicates the existence of an unconscious institutional defence against the acknowledgement of work-related stress. There seems to be an irrational reluctance to look at the costs of stress in work settings for fear that to acknowledge something is only to make it worse.

ELEMENTS IN STAFF GROUP FACILITATION

Assessing the initial request by way of an initial consultation

I was asked to consult to a group of staff in a unit. Six months before this a new consultant to the unit had been appointed, resulting in a tremendous row between the consultant and key members of staff, some of whom had already left; others served notice of their intention to leave.

At the first meeting, I introduced myself. I mentioned three things about myself. These were: who I was, what my job title was, and something about my experience with groups. I was particularly interested to see which parts of my identity seemed to register with them. They made no real response to my introduction and this left me with a sense that they were too preoccupied to pay much attention to me at this stage. I then mentioned how it was I came to be meeting with them. I asked them if it was correct to assume that this was with their agreement. I explained that our meeting was a consultation, a time for questions and exploration of issues concerning their request rather than the first meeting of a staff support group. I did not tell them anything of what I had already been told, hence I was asked a question about what I already knew. I responded that being briefed about the group was not the kind of information I found useful. I was there to learn from them what they thought the issues were. I tried to find neutral words such as 'issues' rather than use terms such as 'problems' or 'difficulties', so as to not feed the group with my undigested presuppositions. My purpose was to gather first-hand information of what they thought, felt, and were able to say.

I began to note my own internal reactions to being with this group. I felt anxious and nervous, as if I had to try to find a solution to the obvious distress I was picking up. I felt frightened by feeling so responsible. I felt if I put a foot wrong, powerful anger would focus on me. I noticed how the staff related to each other and my first impression was of three principal associations. The consultant, senior registrar, and registrar represented the medical profile. There was the group who had found the consultant's arrival so traumatic. There was a third group made up of two students, a newly appointed therapist, a recently appointed senior nurse practitioner, and the unit administrator. After a while I noticed that the senior registrar and registrar associated themselves more with this third group. This group seemed to adopt a neutral position. I was reminded of sensitive children who know something terrible has happened between the parents in the secrecy of the bedroom. This group seemed both curious but also careful not to want to know too much. Taking sides was not going to be helpful. From my own reactions I speculated on their fear of getting entangled in the mess. Neither they nor I wanted to get too close to the mess. Despite attempts to be thoughtful and reflective, the protagonists could not hide the real anger and pain they felt towards each other. There was an entrenched belief that this was all someone's fault. The disagreement seemed to be about whose.

Part of assessing the initial request will involve listening to what the staff team is asking for, and determining whether this can be reasonably responded to. However, staff teams will not always be able to say, or even to know, what it is they want. Often what they do say easily reveals powerful, almost magical expectations of the group and the facilitator. Theoretically, a staff group is a necessary tool for any team whose work requires sophisticated levels of collaboration around the work task. However, the facilitator needs to be able to assess whether there are enough of the basic dynamic and constituent ingredients for a group to be a viable tool for this staff team. The following questions might usefully be posed: What seem to be the expectations of what a facilitated support group will achieve? If these seem high does the team show an ability to moderate them in response to the facilitator's comments? Does the strength of commitment to a possible group from all sections of the team exceed the threshold for viability? Is there too much anxiety for there to be a reasonable expectation for the development of a working alliance?

By the end of this consultation I was able to make some suggestions based upon my experience of them over sixty minutes. I told them that I did not believe this situation could be repaired. I carefully watched their reaction. I felt they were relieved by my comment. I suggested the present process of separation be completed, at which point it might then be useful to institute a staff support group. Anxiety at this point rose in the group. One person asked what would be the point in that? In my reply I attempted to link three of my perceptions together in the form of a working hypothesis. Firstly, my own feelings of discomfort and concern for my own survival told me that feelings of anger, hurt, and the desire to blame others were presently too high to be worked with. Secondly, despite the need of some in the consultation to believe otherwise, I believed that the roots of this conflict lay outside a simple clash of personalities. I explained that I believed that the origin of conflict that degenerates into an intractable personality clash is a focusing of tensions experienced from the work and the surrounding institutional–social environment. Thirdly, if my interpretation was correct, although the present situation could be managed by malcontented members of the team leaving, unless this were accompanied by the development of understanding about what had taken place, the unconscious causes of the present breakdown would be likely to reconstellate around some future point of tension in the team. The purpose of this working hypothesis was for me to try to offer them some reflection on what I had experienced of them around their central concerns, and, at the same time, to assess the capacity for psychological thinking in the group.

My third point was taken up and a brief discussion of what I meant then took place. I suggested that we finish the consultation and that they should take time and then confirm whether they wanted to proceed with forming a staff support group and whether I was what they were looking for in a facilitator. One person looked puzzled and said that she did not understand my last statement: had it not already been agreed to start a group – so what was I talking about?

The facilitator

Many staff group facilitators have undergone training in group therapy. Some may have a training in institutional consultation. Within health care institutional settings, facilitators will usually have a background either in some branch of psychology or in one or other of the key caring professions. Backgrounds vary, but two elements are common.

Firstly, the facilitator must have had experience of being in groups. Most useful is having been a member of a type of group which is sometimes called an 'experiential group', sometimes a 'training group'. My own approach to groups is psychodynamic, and therefore to work with staff support groups in the way I outline here requires experience and theoretical knowledge about the unconsious processes that influence group dynamics. While training is important, so too is good life experience in institutional and work-based group cultures.

Secondly, the facilitator must be able to tolerate doubt and the uncertainty of being in a continual state of not knowing. Bion characterized this as ridding oneself of memory and desire (Bion, 1987). However, trying to be Bion in a staff support group is an arid experience for all concerned. Each person must find their own identity with regard to style. Psychodynamic psychology offers tools for understanding, and guidelines for safe and containing practice. One's own motivation for this work is an important qualification. As a chaplain, working with staff support groups is particularly relevant to the exercise of my pastoral concern for the healthy functioning of institutional life in the hospital where I work. My style results from the integration of my pastoral identity with my psychodynamic group understanding and training. This particularly attunes me to the relationship between the way we manage work-related stress and the quality of care given to those entrusted to our care. Good quality of care cannot be delivered by an institution that neglects its own corporate health.

Interpretation

In a therapy group, interpretations are directed towards making conscious the unconscious processes of the members of the group. The business of this group is its members. They do not encounter one another except in the setting of the group. Interpretations in an experiential learning group tend to be directed towards making conscious the group's unconscious processes. The business of this group is the group itself and its recognition of group processes. The business of the staff group is not its members, not even the group, it is the culture surrounding the work. Interpretation must, therefore, be directed towards an analysis of the work culture as reflected in the dynamics of interaction between members in the group (Menzies Lyth, 1989).

> I facilitated over a period of some time a staff group on a unit where the work related closely to anxiety experienced between mothers and infants. In the time I had been working with the group I had seen two nurse managers leave the unit in unhappy circumstances. With arrival of a third manager I was concerned whether the pattern would be repeated. Around each of the previous two leavings, interpretations by me had made little impact on the nurses. When faced with a period of conflict between the third manager and the nursing team, my interpretations met with some acceptance in the team. How do I account for this change?

Anyone is likely to retreat into a kind of dysfunctional behaviour when under stress. Stress also causes the staff team to behave collectively in a dysfunctional manner. If it can be looked at it can be seen that dysfunction in the leader and dysfunction in the team are reflections of key elements of the internal dysfunction within the patients. In the situation of a breakdown between nurse manager and nursing team, all three elements will be present. However, on the first occasion of facing this situation, I was dominated by feelings about the manager and the way she was responding to the difficulties in the team. The nurses indulged in a kind of therapeutic style of interpretation of their manager's behaviour. I suspect my interpretations were influenced by this, no matter how hard I tried not to be personal. On the second occasion, my feelings about the lethal qualities of the group came to the fore. My interpretations were aimed at what the group appeared to be doing to the manager. In each instance I theoretically knew that both situations were rooted in the dynamics of the work. However, I seemed dominated by my feelings, with the result that I directed interpretations at the wrong level of experience. On the third occasion I directed my interpretations to the relationship between what was happening within the team and the anxieties projected from the type of work performed on the unit. I found myself commenting more upon the dynamics of the mother who finds herself both responsible for and yet in a form of primitive competition with her infant. Interpretations directed to this level of the unit's experience helped the members of the team to begin to recognize and reflect upon a pattern which, once traced and located in the work, could be understood rather than acted upon. The facilitator must develop an internal resonance with their interpretation. Knowing the truth about something is not the same as finding the place within oneself from which that truth resonates in an interpretation.

Interpretation is a way for the facilitator to help the group to understand the way it is unconsciously influenced by processes over which it exercises no control. These processes are detected in attitudes, assumptions, and practices which characterize relations between the different members of the team and between the team and the environment. While listening to what is said (the content) the facilitator works at trying to learn what the purpose of the discussion taking place might be (the process). Interesting and always potentially alluring though content often is, the question for the facilitator is: what might the purpose of this discussion be in relation to anxieties around the work or institutional setting? I want to emphasize that the facilitator does not possess clairvoyance. The facilitator's only tool is a developed capacity to observe, digest, and reprocess the group's unconscious communications into words that can be heard and understood.

Boundaries

An important factor in both therapy and experiential groups is that the members are there by voluntary agreement. The members of the staff support group are present by virtue of belonging to the team. The difficulty is that the team is not usually coterminous with the staff group. This makes for a permeable boundary as the constituency of the group is in a constant state of ebb and flux due to shift work patterns and staff turnover. Therefore, the group is constantly preoccupied with the behaviour of team members who are not present in the group. This is a difficult issue. I have heard it said that if the consultant will not attend the group then there is no point having one. But in my experience it is an exception for the consultant to attend a staff support group, though this seems less of an issue as younger generations of doctors take up consultant posts. Preoccupation with non-attenders may be a legitimate concern of a staff group. It can also mean that the energy of the group keeps seeping out through a hole in the side of its boundary wall.

> The staff in one group frequently approached a near mutinous state caused by their anger at the consultant's refusal to attend the group. In their dissatisfaction with him they began to treat me as if I could be their champion against him. In their imagination, unlike him, I came and listened and appeared understanding. Despite the existence of this weekly group, the consultant arranged a team day for the unit. To protest, the nurses threatened to lock themselves in the seclusion room. They seemed very put out by my not having been invited to attend, if not lead, this team day. This was communicated to the consultant, who eventually asked to meet me privately. During this meeting he had the opportunity to discover that my becoming an alternative leader was a projection of the nurses who had felt abandoned by him. He then invited me to the team day. The nurses were surprised when I declined to go, explaining that my relationship to the unit could only be conducted through the staff support group for as long as I was its facilitator. Some weeks after this meeting we had a consultation with all the disciplines attending. This resulted in the consultant attending the weekly group. The group was very pleased with this, but it presented them with another dilemma. It was easy to bemoan his absence, but they now had to do something with his presence. His attendance has over time robbed them of one less defence against having to work with issues more constructively and take responsibility for effecting changes.

A USEFUL METAPHOR

James Mather (1976) offers a description of the different functions of the motor neuron and nervous systems in the human body by way of an analogy to social and institutional structures designed for task organization and stress monitoring. He concludes that, whereas in the human being the motor neuron system is simple and develops relatively quickly, most time in the human physical development process is given over to the development of the complex nervous system. This system monitors the stress and cost to the body of motor and muscular activity through a multiplicity of communicative neuron arches connecting the two systems. In social institutions the exact reverse is the case. Here the nervous system equivalent is much less developed. Social organization expends most time and energy in task performance. Priority is given to organization that serves this end. There is often no separation between command and communication systems. Thus hierarchical command structures distort and inhibit communication gathering systems. Consequently, in social organizations there is little developed communication structure capable of independently monitoring the stress and cost exacted on the workers in task performace. This is equivalent to the brain silencing the nervous system's registration of pain as a warning against impending physiological damage. The body can behave in this way, but only in response to a life threat. Life in our institutions is stressful because the absence of communciation and stress monitoring organization pushes collective functioning into adrenalin mode for unsustainable periods of time. This produces the metaphorical equivalent of constant muscle tearing and bone breaking within the fabric of our institutional life.

The staff support group is an instrument that belongs to a range of instruments designed to monitor and collect information about the collective stress-producing processes affecting work culture. The staff support group is diagnostic rather than instrumental. Its purpose is to provide a series of snapshots of a team's collective functioning at a given point of time. This information forms the basis of a diagnosis. Diagnosis is not treatment, but treatment without efficient diagnosis is ineffective. The central question to be answered is: do we really want to know the costs of professional stress? The answer might mean having to change the way we do things.

REFERENCES

Bion, W.R. (1987) *Experience in Groups and Other Papers*, Tavistock Publications, London.

Mather, J. (1976) A brain of brains. *Contact: The Interdisciplinary Journal of Pastoral Studies*, **97**, 3.

Menzies Lyth, I. (1988) *Containing Anxiety in Institutions*, vol. 1, Free Association Books, London.

Menzies Lyth, I. (1989) *The Dynamics of the Social*, Free Association Books, London.

Stress management interventions

12

Jerome Carson and Elizabeth Kuipers

INTRODUCTION

There is accumulating research evidence of the stressful nature of the health and social care professions. A recent review of stress in mental health professionals (Carson and Fagin, 1996) presented evidence concerning stress in occupational therapists (Sweeney and Nichols, 1996), psychiatrists (Deary, Agius and Sadler, 1996), social workers (Pottage and Huxley, 1996), clinical psychologists (Cushway and Tyler, 1996), mental health nurses (Fagin et al., 1996), and case managers and community psychiatric teams (Oliver and Kuipers, 1996). Neither have general nurses (e.g. Hipwell, Tyler and Wilson, 1989) or doctors (Firth-Cozens, 1987) been immune from this research trend. While it seems intuitively appealing to state that stressed carers may not provide the most nurturing care, empirical demonstrations of this supposed truism are hard to find. From the professional's point of view, conceptual models of stress and possible effects on patient care are probably of secondary importance to the issue of what can be done to reduce their own stress levels, reduce burnout, and improve coping skills. Work-based stress management seeks to reduce the pressures on professionals, and is the issue that we address in this chapter.

Rather like the field of stress itself, 'stress management' is an umbrella term. It encompasses a wide range of different methods designed principally to reduce stress and improve coping abilities. In this review we begin by presenting an overview of the field. We then consider what stress managers can learn from their participants to enhance their programmes. Following this we examine a range of work-based stress management interventions reported in the research literature. We then critically appraise the work in this area and make suggestions for future research.

STRESS MANAGEMENT AT WORK: AN OVERVIEW

Ross and Altmaier (1994) provide a helpful overview of the work stress management field. They divide interventions into two main categories. Firstly *individual interventions* and secondly *workplace interventions*. They suggest that the former can be further subdivided into strategies that are primarily preventive or primarily combative.

Individual interventions

Preventive strategies are responses to alleviate stress as it is initially perceived. They fall into four categories:

(1) *Monitoring stressors and symptoms.* This includes stress diaries, muscle monitoring, and the use of tension thermometers.
(2) *Marshalling resources and attacking stressors.* Here they include social skills, assertion training, and problem-solving skills training.
(3) *Tolerating stressors.* These cover cognitive appraisal, cognitive restructuring, cognitive rehearsal, and stress innoculation training.
(4) *Lowering arousal.* Here they mention a whole range of methods such as breathing, muscular relaxation, transcendental meditation, the Benson technique, etc. This last is a meditative technique with four main elements: being in a quiet environment; having an object to dwell upon, either gazing at a symbol or repeating a word or sound; having a passive attitude, emptying thoughts and distractions from the mind; being in a comfortable position that the individual can remain in for around 20 minutes (Benson and Klipper, 1982).

Combative strategies fall into three main areas :

(1) *Developing coping resources.* This includes social support and time management.
(2) *Altering stress-inducing behaviour patterns.* Changing type A behaviour patterns, for instance (Cartwright and Cooper, 1997).
(3) *Avoiding stressors through adjustment.* Individuals need to consider their family/work balance, and also career planning. Combative strategies are for dealing with stressors that are already happening.

Workplace interventions

Not surprisingly, workplace interventions are quite different in focus. Broadly they fit into six main areas according to Ross and Altmaier:

(1) *Role characteristics.* Reducing work stress through tackling issues such as job ambiguity, work overload and underload, and changing expectations.

(2) *Job characteristics.* Reducing stress by job redesign, job enrichment, or job enlargement.

(3) *Interpersonal relationships.* Improving communication methods and systems at work.

(4) *Organizational structure and climate.* Encouraging decentralization, greater participation in decision making, and surveying work-force attitudes.

(5) *Human resource management systems.* There are a whole series of personnel management functions that may help reduce stress at work; for instance, recruitment and selection policies that select staff that are likely to fit in well with existing teams. Staff appraisal systems may also help.

(6) *Physical qualities.* It may be necessary to change the quality of the work environment.

Our concern in this chapter is clearly more with individual stress management based approaches, which are in fact much better evaluated than are organizational approaches (Murphy, 1988; Cox, 1993). However, as Martin (1992) points out, there is a distinct danger that such approaches may 'blame the victim of stress … without any attention to … work rules, supervisory policies, lack of benefits, the work environment or the employing organization' (p. 207).

Cooper (1996) sees workplace interventions as fitting into a primary, secondary, or tertiary prevention model. In the *primary* prevention of workplace stress the aim is to reduce or eliminate stressors and positively to promote a supportive and healthy work environment. Stress audits can enable organizations to monitor stress levels in employees. *Secondary* prevention is concerned with prompt detection and management of depression and anxiety by increasing self-awareness and improving stress management skills. The aim here is to help workers evaluate the psychological effects of stress and to develop their own personal stress control plans. *Tertiary* prevention is concerned with the rehabilitation and recovery process of those individuals who have suffered or are suffering from stress-related disorders. The main forms of help here are workplace counselling and employee assistance programmes. The majority of work stress management programmes focus at the secondary level, though the Louisville programme, described later, is an exception to this.

Stress management interventions often include the following :

- Changing, increasing, or enhancing coping responses and resources.
- Teaching arousal reduction techniques such as relaxation.
- Changing perceptions or appraisals of work stressors via cognitive restructuring (Dollard and Winefield, 1996).

CONTRIBUTIONS FROM STAFF RESEARCH TO STRESS MANAGEMENT PROGRAMMES

Stress management research often makes an implicit assumption that the trainers know best how to manage and avoid stress. Trainees or participants are often viewed as passive victims of stress, though some workers have a more collaborative approach (Martin, 1992). Before starting any intervention it is important to investigate any literature on the presence and management of particular stresses specific to the professional group being worked with.

Sweeney interviewed 30 qualified occupational therapists and asked how they coped with stress (Sweeney, Nichols and Cormack, 1993). From these interviews she was able to recommend a number of strategies that individual occupational therapists could utilize to help them cope with stress at work. She suggested the following :

(1) Taking time out during the working day for coffee and lunch breaks, preferably in non-treatment settings.
(2) Programming some time each day as non-treatment time, e.g. for report writing.
(3) Having a cut-off point at the end of each day to indicate the transition from a work to a social role; an exercise class could serve this function.
(4) Spacing out rewarding and non-rewarding tasks.
(5) Using positive coping skills in the workplace, such as time management, prioritizing and limit setting.
(6) Cultivating personal awareness of stress as well as discussing stress issues with colleagues.

Sweeney's suggestions are probably applicable to other professions. In a similar vein, Bunce and West (1994) looked at the use of innovation as a coping strategy with 333 health care professionals. Interestingly one of the examples given by a physiotherapist in this study was to see 'the difficult children as early as possible in the day when I'm at my best' (p. 325). The importance of this approach is that it highlights the ability of individual professionals to change workplace stressors as well as themselves.

Just as studying how coping strategies may help staff (Koeske, Kirk and Koeske, 1993), it may also be useful to examine specific stressors confronting different professional groups. Sweeney has developed a measure of occupational stress for occupational therapists (Sweeney, Nichols and Kline, 1991), and at least two groups of researchers have developed specific measures of stress in general nurses (Grey-Toft and Anderson, 1981; Harris, 1989). Carson and his colleagues have developed two self-report measures for assessing stress in mental health nurses. On the CPN Stress Questionnaire (Brown *et al.*, 1995), the three greatest stressors for community mental health nurses were found to be :

(1) Not having facilities in the community that you can refer clients to.

(2) Knowing that there are likely to be long waiting lists before clients can get access to services.
(3) Having to deal with suicidal clients on your own.

These stressors have clear implications for management (see Carson *et al.*, 1995, for a fuller discussion of this). For instance, if we examine the third stressor on the list, it is clear that the possibility of a client committing suicide is always present in mental health work. Training in how to assess the risk of suicide in clients and in what to do next, is crucial, as is being able to discuss the issues openly. As community mental health nurses often see clients on their own in the community, it is critical for them to be able to discuss potentially suicidal clients with colleagues in team meetings, reviews, or informally, with opportunities to discuss their reactions to any incident that might occur. In contrast to this, Fagin *et al.* (1996) found that the top three stressors for ward-based mental health nurses were :

(1) Inadequate staffing cover, leading to potentially dangerous situations.
(2) Dealing with changes in the health service and hospital closures.
(3) Low morale and poor atmosphere within the organization.

The first stressor was found to be the top rated in four separate hospitals. Clearly this is an issue for hospital managers who set staffing budgets. There is obviously a pay-off between running a cost-effective service and a safe one. The development of a body of empirical knowledge for specific professional groups will help us to develop stress management packages tailored to the needs of each particular profession. In the next section we describe specific stress management interventions that have been used with health and social care professionals. This review is intended to be illustrative and not exhaustive.

SPECIFIC STRESS MANAGEMENT INTERVENTIONS

Bradley (1992) describes stress and time management workshops for social work students. Participants were initially asked to define stress, then to recognize individual symptoms, moving on to a discussion of personality and levels of stress. Attitudes and beliefs about caring were also considered. Relaxation, leisure, exercise, and diet were examined as ways of coping. The morning section of the workshop ended with a discussion of burnout, and small groups then brainstormed how burnout could be avoided. The afternoon of the workshop focused on time management. The author's own experience from field settings was that 'those who were more organized on a day-to-day basis, who were clear about priorities, who handled one job at a time, were more likely to be successful and less likely to take sick leave' (p. 12). Students were taught to set goals, to learn how to prioritize and, most importantly, how to get started on the process. The workshop ended with an audio tape of breathing and relaxation exercises, followed by a brief guided fantasy. This sort of stress workshop is no doubt typical of thousands of similar courses run in many settings. As the author herself concludes, evaluation was based solely on 'soft' data, with no empirical evidence presented of the workshop's efficacy.

In a study of mental health nurses, Kunkler and Whittick (1991) found it almost impossible to recruit nurses to participate in their stress management workshops. For instance the third workshop they ran was attended by a single participant, forcing them to offer individual rather than group sessions. They suggest that for mental health nurses, 'Attendance may ... be interpreted as a sign of weakness' (p. 176). Our own clinical experience confirms this impression.

In a more scientific study of stress management, Freedy and Hobfoll (1994) assigned female general nurses to one of two interventions. The first of these was a dual resource intervention comprising social support and mastery, the second a single resource intervention, targeting only enhancement of mastery. The mastery condition comprised five weekly 75 minute sessions of stress innoculation training (Meichenbaum, 1985). There were 49 nurses in the dual resource condition and 38 in the single resource condition. The authors found greater improvement in the dual resource groups. The study does unfortunately have a number of methodological flaws, such as having only a five-week follow-up, not having random allocation of individual participants, and providing insufficient detail about the social support intervention to enable its proper evaluation.

A third example of a stress management programme is provided by Michie and Sandhu (1994). They describe optional groups in stress management that were offered to medical students at a major London teaching hospital. The intervention comprised only three two-hour sessions conducted over consecutive weeks. Groups of ten medical students were taught about the nature of stress, its causes and consequences, and how to reduce high levels of stress and prevent its buildup. Homework tasks encouraged students to try out the techniques and to plan their own stress management programme. Only 19 out of 111 medical students chose to enrol on the programme. Attenders were more anxious, less satisfied with themselves and their life, and perceived their work and outside functioning to be poorer. However, non-attenders became more dissatisfied at work and outside over a one-year follow-up period, whereas course attenders showed no such deterioration. The authors suggest that stress management may provide long-term benefits. Despite these encouraging findings, there is a need to conduct a proper randomized controlled trial, as this was only a preliminary, though successful, first study.

Long and Flood (1993) review the evidence that exercise can be a helpful method of combating work stress. The rationale behind using exercise as a form of stress management is the claim that consistent aerobic exercise will improve physical fitness. Improving physical fitness will then, it is assumed, lead to better mental health outcomes. This is the old adage of a healthy mind in a healthy body (*mens sana in corpore sano*). Long and Flood suggest that employees 'who are the least fit and have the greatest room for improvement are likely to benefit most from an exercise programme that challenges them' (p. 114). They further point out that exercise is best taught as an emotion-focused coping strategy (Lazarus and

Folkman, 1984). Jex (1991), presents a more critical assessment of the value of exercise in reducing work stress. He argues that there are few controls for differences between 'exercisers' and 'non-exercisers'. Individuals with 'high levels of self-motivation and optimism, low levels of negative affectivity, and internal locus of control, will be more likely to exercise consistently' (p. 143). These personality factors may have a stronger impact on stress outcomes than exercise alone. Indeed this was exemplified by an exercise study that used well motivated MBA students as participants (Kerr and Vlaswinkel, 1995). Because exercise is less stigmatizing, it may be especially acceptable to health and social care professionals as an intervention strategy, but its role in improving mental health outcomes requires further evaluation (Glenister, 1996).

Another technique that is commonly employed as a form of stress management is assertiveness training. Lee and Crockett (1994) describe a randomized controlled trial of assertiveness training versus a control condition comprising 'updated knowledge of new technology on computer applications in nursing'. Participants received six two-hour workshops over a two-week period, with a further two weeks of follow-up. Both samples were found to be 'subassertive' and experiencing high levels of stress. By the end of training and at follow-up, the assertiveness training group reported significantly lower levels of stress and higher levels of assertiveness. However, it would have been more informative to have compared the assertiveness training against a more credible stress management intervention than the one utilized in this study. The follow-up period was also too short to evaluate significant effects.

Hyman (1993) describes a multi-component stress management package that was delivered via three three-hour sessions. The programme covered a range of areas including team building, communication skills, and self-esteem. Stress management techniques included breathing exercises, guided visualization, and a 'shoulder massage with a partner'. The workshops were attended by 188 staff, but Hyman chose only to conduct evaluations on 51 participants, 'a stratified random sample'. Hyman used the Maslach Burnout Inventory (Maslach and Jackson, 1986) and a six-item work atmosphere scale developed specifically for the project. Participants were given the questionnaires after they had attended the workshops in a 'retrospective pretest design'. They completed one set of questionnaires rating their attitudes 'today', and the second rating their attitudes 'then', in this instance before they attended the workshops. Hyman found significant improvements in personal accomplishment, lower emotional exhaustion, and lower (but not significantly so) depersonalization scores on the Maslach Scale. Attenders also rated their work atmosphere as being significantly improved. Qualitative comments backed this up. Hyman acknowledges the weakness of the retrospective design, but was forced to adopt this as she was only able to conduct the evaluations once the workshops had commenced.

In one of the best designed stress management intervention studies, Snow and Kline (1995) conducted a randomized controlled trial with 239 female clerical workers from four different work locations. The intervention group received 15

90-minute stress management sessions. These covered a range of issues, such as dealing with multiple roles, identifying stressful situations, problem solving, managing stress, communication skills, personal networks and social support, rethinking the problem, and a personal stress management plan. Impressively, participants were assessed both before and after intervention and at six and 22 months follow-up. The authors used a range of measures covering stressors, coping, social support, and stress outcomes. While the intervention group differed on seven measures at six months follow-up (e.g. they showed less avoidance coping and less alcohol use), by 22 months there was only one difference – fewer somatic symptoms in the intervention group. In terms of the types of study conducted in the work stress field, this study is better than most. It is perhaps strongest in the clinical measurement aspects, yet weakest on the organizational side. It would have been intriguing to learn the pattern of sickness absence of the two groups. Did the intervention group take fewer days off sick as a result of the intervention? Similarly, did the intervention group have stronger organizational commitment and higher morale as a result of the stress management programme? Finally, although this study was not conducted with health or social care professionals, its robust design provides us with a good example of a well conducted intervention study.

A final programme to be described is that of the Louisville Medical School. Students are introduced to health awareness in a voluntary four-day course before the start of their studies. Interestingly, in contrast to the programme described by Michie and Sandhu (1994), more than 90 per cent of students enrol in this programme. The programme can be truly described as holistic. Benor (1995) describes its components as including :

(1) *Using second-year students as health tutors.* Second-year students share their anxieties and coping styles for dealing with the stresses of medical training. Tutors meet daily during the programme with 10–15 new students, and then periodically during the first year.
(2) *The importance of healthy eating.* Breakfast is prepared by second-year tutors for the first three days, and on the last day by the new students. The emphasis is on 'doing'. Lectures are given on healthy diets, with a focus on assessing the fat content of meals.
(3) *Helpful publications.* A range of publications is provided including a cookbook (with nutritional guidelines), the *Medical Student Unauthorised Survival Handbook*, and *Steps to Good Health*. The importance of relaxation time for 'emotional and intellectual refuelling in order to increase productivity' is repeatedly emphasized.
(4) *Supportive medical school policies.* Students are encouraged to cooperate in collaborative note taking and are actively discouraged from competition.
(5) *Encouragement of intellectual and creative pursuits.* The pursuit of intellectual and recreational activities outside of medicine is actively encouraged. This is taught in the course through demonstration, lectures, and experiential presentations.

(6) *Problems facing medical schools*. Problems of alcohol and substance abuse in doctors as well as issues around sexuality were covered. A minister stressed the importance of spiritual development. An experiential demonstration of tai chi was also given.

(7) *Ethical issues and professional personal attitudes*. This section tackled issues such as sexual harassment and prejudice.

(8) *Stress management through exercise*. This was a major focus of the programme, with much encouragement and opportunity to participate in daily athletics activities.

Support groups for students from non-science backgrounds, married, single parents, etc. are also provided.

We are aware of no empirical data to suggest that medical students exposed to the Louisville programme are in fact less stressed than medical students from other medical schools, but the originators of this programme are to be praised for their efforts to ensure that the issue of stress management permeates all aspects of the doctors' training. Other health and social care professionals might do well to emulate this approach.

There is no definitive evidence as to which components of stress management training work best. However, as Rosch stated (Rosch, 1994, p. 221), 'Just as stress differs for each of us, no stress reduction technique works for everyone. Regular meditation, jogging and autogenic training work fine for some, but when arbitrarily imposed on others may actually prove stressful. Similarly few fixed stress management training programmes are optimal for all circumstances.' Equally, it is critical not to overlook organizational aspects of stress management (Dollard and Winefield, 1996).

A CRITICAL APPRAISAL OF THE STRESS MANAGEMENT FIELD

Briner and Reynolds (1993) criticize a great deal of the occupational stress research, which often assumes that almost all work problems are the result of excessive stress at work. They argue that 'new theories must be better grounded, and sophisticated enough to account for the richness and complexity of human behaviour'. This is despite the fact that some theoretically grounded work does exist (Roger and Hudson, 1995). In a second paper, Reynolds and Briner (1994) suggest that '... occupational stress reduction is ... one of the many fads initiated by academics, commercialised by consultants and embraced by managers but that ultimately fail to deliver the panacea-like solutions which they promise' (p. 75). They also point to the paradox of increasing stress management training in the absence of data on the efficacy of these approaches. They argue that the majority of interventions focus on individuals, rather than on changing aspects of the work environment that are commercially unattractive. Managers and employers, they believe, are more likely to be supportive of interventions that focus on the employee and 'which do not involve any meaningful or disruptive organizational level response' (p. 81).

Among their criticisms, Reynolds and Briner (1994) state that several studies in the work stress field report distress levels similar to those of the normal population. Hence, they argue, most of the employees enrolling in stress management programmes may not be suffering from clinical levels of distress. They describe it thus: 'stress management training provides healthy, non-distressed employees with a range of strategies and techniques which they can use to manage work demands' (p. 78). However, ethical constraints make it difficult to avoid this issue. For instance if only employees with very high General Health Questionnaire scores are considered to have a sufficient level of distress, this would mean only including those with scores above 10 to be comparable with patient samples (Carson and Brewerton, 1991). Relating this criterion to our research with mental health nurses shows that only about 10 per cent of the 648 nurses surveyed would score in this range (Fagin et al., 1996). Persuading this 10 per cent to enter into a randomized controlled trial might well be difficult and cause problems of stigma. Even if it were possible to allocate, say, 100 nurses to a stress mangement intervention, with a further 100 receiving some control condition, this would involve a survey of 2000 nurses. Clearly this is not feasible unless adequate screening and resources were available. An alternative might be to offer intervention only to those who were already asking for counselling, as this might indicate sufficient distress, but of course self-selection would make this an oddly biased sample and would have to be controlled for.

FUTURE DEVELOPMENTS IN STRESS MANAGEMENT RESEARCH

Theory–practice links

It is difficult not to agree with Briner and Reynolds (1993) that the bulk of stress management interventions have a weak theoretical base. Few of the studies described earlier were well grounded theoretically, apart from that of Snow and Kline (1995). Before intervening in any clinical problem, we need to have a good understanding of the scope of the problem. As clinical psychologists we tend to be best at individual assessment and treatment, but not at understanding organizational aspects of the stress process. Thus the question arises: what sort of model should guide stress management intervention work? Most workers now accept that a transactional model (Cox, 1978), sometimes also called a stress-appraisal-coping model (Lazarus, 1995), best accounts for the existing data on stress. We have developed our own version of this model for understanding the process of stress in mental health nurses, but it could also be applied to other health and social care professions.

Our revised model of the stress process (Fagin et al., 1996) has three major components. Firstly it suggests that stressors come from three major *external sources*. There are specific occupational stressors. We outlined earlier the three top stressors for mental health nurses. For instance, for community mental health nurses the third most stressful aspect of the job was 'dealing with suicidal clients on your own'. These occupational stressors will probably vary depending on the unique stresses facing each professional group. In Britain, social workers have considerable statutory responsibilities, which cause additional stress to many social workers (Gibson, McGrath and Reid, 1989; Jones, Fletcher and Ibbetson, 1991). Sweeney has demonstrated that occupational therapists experience a lot of stress related to their professional self-esteem (Sweeney, Nichols and Kline, 1991). The second source of external stress comes from hassles or uplifts (Kanner *et al.*, 1981). These are minor everyday events that can have a cumulative effect, such as having a difficult journey to work, or poor back-up at work. These are not major stressors on their own, but taken together can cause considerable irritation and distress. The final source of external stress comes from major life events. The importance of life events has been well known and researched since the seminal work of Holmes and Rahe (1967). Clearly, staff going through major life transitions, such as divorce or bereavement, may have difficulties functioning at optimum efficiency. Professionals are said to be able to leave their personal problems at home and not to allow them to interfere with their work but this is unlikely to be true, as there is no evidence that professionals are immune to the effects of major life stressors.

The second major component of our stress model is that of *mediating or buffering* factors. We argue that there are a number of factors that can mediate or buffer the effects of stress. We identify seven such factors in our model, though there may well be more. High levels of self-esteem (Turner and Roszell, 1994), good social support networks (Brugha, 1995), hardiness (Kobassa and Puccetti, 1983), good coping skills (Carver, Scheier and Weintraub, 1989), mastery and personal control (Pearlin *et al.*, 1981), emotional stability (Eysenck and Eysenck, 1975), and good physiological release mechanisms can all serve to minimize the effects of stress on individuals. Physiological release mechanisms cover a range of skills such as the ability to relax, taking regular exercise, having a sense of humour, and the ability to let off steam. We suggest that individuals with these attributes will be better able to deal with the effects of stress than those without them.

The third and final component of our model is that of *stress outcomes*. We divide these into positive stress outcomes, such as psychological health and high job satisfaction, and negative stress outcomes, such as psychological ill health, burnout, and low job satisfaction.

Components of this model now need to be tested. For instance, is it possible to have good job satisfaction yet poor psychological health? Our model suggests not, partly as it builds on the well established research literature that shows burnout to be negatively correlated with job satisfaction (Schaufeli, Enzman and Girault, 1993). Researchers conducting stress management interventions have often intervened using either individual components from our list of mediating or buffering factors, or else two or three of these components in combination. We have suggested that there are seven such factors. A stress management intervention that focuses on all these components should theoretically be more effective. Indeed, we have just completed a randomized controlled trial of social support versus feedback only, in a stress management study with mental health nurses. Follow-up data on this study are not yet available. A second intervention will target all seven mediating or buffering factors in another randomized trial.

In summary, we need to develop and test stress management interventions that are better grounded in theory.

Stress in the caring professions

Work-based stress management interventions tend not to discriminate between the groups to which the interventions are applied. Cox (1993) states that the majority of stress management studies have been targeted more at white collar and managerial workers than blue collar workers. Do stress management interventions work equally well in different settings, i.e. would a stress management intervention developed and applied with a group of factory workers be equally useful with a group of health or social care professionals? The literature reviewed earlier suggests that intervention should take account of specific stresses connected to particular jobs, and the whole burnout literature has been developed from the premise that working in the caring professions creates specific stressors (Maslach, 1993; Leiter and Harvie, 1996). It ought to be noted, however, that there is no single agreed model of the 'burnout' process, which is a rather vaguely described concept. Richardsen and Burke (1995) describe three models and the interventions that derive from their premises. Stress management interventions for health and social care professionals clearly need to be addressed to the particular pressures of working in the caring professions.

There is, however, real evidence of a reluctance by health and social care professionals to recognize that occupational stress is a problem for them. For instance, Walsh, Nichols and Cormack (1991) argued that clinical psychologists were able to identify such problems in their patients and colleagues but were reluctant to consider their own self-care needs. Interestingly, the British Psychological Society's Division of Clinical Psychology focuses on the issue of work stress in their Professional Practice Guidelines (DCP, 1995, p. 39): 'Clinical psychologists need to ensure that they actively pursue a lifestyle and a method and style of working which safeguards fitness to practise. Those working alone, and those with excess work demands and inadequate support, may lack opportunities to protect their capacity to maintain professional standards.' They further state (p. 40) 'Clinical psychologists who are experiencing high levels of personal distress because of either home-based or work-related difficulties, or both, have a duty to seek support and guidance to explore ways to resolve distress appropriately, if their fitness to practise is being impaired.' It remains to be seen whether such principles will actually filter down into practice.

It is undeniable that in Britain stress levels within health and social care professions have risen and are rising. There is also the problem that interventions must be continually updated because of political changes, new legislation, or economic factors such as unemployment. Interventions in the 1990s are obviously going to be different from those in the 1950s or in 2020. While patients' problems may not have changed clinically, their expectations of services are higher, and government legislation through reforms such as the Patient's Charter has further increased pressure on service providers. We have argued elsewhere (Carson and Fagin, 1996) that 'The health service is therefore beginning to mirror the rest of the economy, where job insecurity is prevalent, and where employees accept the notion that they may become unemployed during part of their working lives or that they will have to change jobs more frequently if these are available.' Hence a certain proportion of the stress facing health and social care professionals is due to organizational changes, and no amount of individual stress management training is going to be able to reduce this. Thus any approach to stress management needs to consider a combination of organizational issues and specific individual intervention if any changes are to be implemented.

Evaluating stress management interventions

Two issues are critical with respect to evaluating stress management interventions. Firstly, there needs to be some attempt to utilize common measurement approaches. This will enable researchers to compare across studies. Secondly, interventions need to be more rigorously evaluated than has been the case to date. This will enable us to discover which approaches work best.

In terms of measuring work stress, many researchers are now following a similar model to that outlined earlier. That is, they are assessing *stressors, measuring mediating or moderating variables* such as personality and demographic factors, and finally assessing *stress outcomes* (referred to as 'strain' by some workers, e.g. Beehr, 1995). (See Broers, Evers and Cooper, 1995, for an example of this approach.) It is important therefore to have standardized measures for each of the three stages. Occupational stressors can be measured by generic scales such as the Sources of Stress Scale (Cooper, Sloan and Williams, 1988), or by specific occupational scales (Dua, 1996). Stress outcomes can be evaluated using measures such as the General Health Questionnaire (Goldberg and Williams, 1988), the Maslach Burnout Inventory (Maslach and Jackson, 1986), and measures of job satisfaction such as the Minnesota Satisfaction Questionnaire (Weiss *et al.*, 1977). It is, however, much harder to decide which personality or demographic factors ought to be monitored. Indeed our own model specifies seven such factors, from self-esteem to coping skills. Snow and Kline (1995) criticize the excessive reliance on self-report measures in the research literature. Few researchers use physiological measures such as blood pressure or catecholamine monitoring (Lester, Nebel and Baum, 1994). More research could and should monitor sickness absence among both stress management participants and their controls, yet surprisingly few do so; see Roger and Hudson (1995) for an exception. While it is important to use both valid and reliable measures of stress, clearly the issue is multifactorial.

The earlier section on specific stress management interventions showed a range of evaluations from simple consumer satisfaction measures to the more comprehensive approach of Snow and Kline (1995). Gordon (1994) visited seven firms in four European countries that ran stress management programmes. The content of programmes, he found, '... was mostly on an ad hoc basis. If something worked (judged by trial and error) it remained' (p. 315). Evaluation of these programmes was almost non-existent. However, without careful evaluation, we are unlikely to discover whether stress management interventions can live up to the promises of their advocates. Cox (1993) argues that there are three main reasons for evaluating stress management programmes. Firstly, to discover if they work. Secondly, to compare both across and within programmes, to see what are the most effective programme components. Thirdly, to assess the cost–benefit or cost effectiveness of programmes.

CONCLUSIONS

In summary, it must be concluded that the jury is still out on stress management training; whilst it seems logical that such interventions should promote employee health, there are not yet sufficient data to be confident that they do.

Cox (1993, p. 73)

When stress reduction programmes are properly designed and implemented, they significantly reduce illness, absenteeism, and employee turnover, and impressively improve productivity and bottom line benefits.

Rosch (1994, p. 221)

These contrasting perspectives of the effectiveness of stress management training demonstrate that much work needs to be done to improve the design, implementation, and evaluation of work-based stress management training. Cooper (1986) may well be correct that the development and evaluation of new programmes will require collaboration between clinical and occupational psychologists. His advice could also be extended to other professions. For instance, behavioural nurse therapists and occupational health nurses might collaborate in developing and evaluating stress management interventions for nurses.

We must, however, be aware of the danger that the provision of stress management might lead to blaming the individual and neglecting the importance of organizational influences on stress (Newton, 1995). The issue of stress management is one that needs to be taken up at a variety of levels, both locally and nationally, and individual programmes are only likely to be helpful if organizational aspects can also be changed. In the USA, the National Institute of Occupational Safety and Health proposed four categories of action to prevent work-related psychological disorders (Sauter, Murphy and Hurrell, 1990):

(1) Job design to improve working conditions.
(2) Surveillance of psychological disorders and risk factors.
(3) Information dissemination, education, and training.
(4) Enrichment of psychological health services for workers.

Stress management programmes have an important part to play in this vision. Stress at work is everyone's business. For too long, health and social care professionals have been reluctant to acknowledge their own stressors. The task ahead is to develop and implement acceptable and cost-effective stress management programmes, both individually and at an organizational level, that are well grounded theoretically, carefully evaluated, and maximally effective.

REFERENCES

Beehr, T. (1995) *Psychological Stress in the Workplace*, Routledge, London.
Benor, D. (1995) The Louisville Programme for medical student health awareness. *Contemporary Therapies in Medicine*, **3**, 93–9.
Benson, H. and Klipper, M. (1982) *The Relaxation Response*. Collins, London.
Bradley, G. (1992) Stress and time management workshops for qualifying social workers. *Social Work Education*, **11** (1), 5–15.
Briner, R. and Reynolds, S. (1993) Bad theory and bad practice in occupational stress. *The Occupational Psychologist*, **19**, 8–13.
Broers, P. Evers, A. and Cooper, C. (1995) Differences in occupational stress in three European countries. *International Journal of Stress Management*, **2** (4), 171–80.
Brown, D. Leary, J. Carson, J. *et al.* (1995) Stress and the community mental health nurse: the development of a measure. *Journal of Psychiatric and Mental Health Nursing*, **2** (1), 9–12.
Brugha, T. (ed.) (1995) *Social Support and Psychiatric Disorder: Research Findings and Guidelines for Clinical Practice*, Cambridge University Press, Cambridge.
Bunce, D. and West, M. (1994) Changing work environments: innovative coping responses to occupational stress. *Work and Stress*, **8** (4), 319–31.
Carson, J. and Brewerton, T. (1991) Out of the clinic into the classroom. *Adults Learning*, **2** (9), 256–7.
Carson, J. and Fagin, L. (1996) Stress in mental health professionals: a cause for concern or an inevitable part of the job. *The International Journal of Social Psychiatry*, **42** (2), 79–81.
Carson, J. Bartlett, H. Brown, D. and Hopkinson, P. (1995) Findings from the qualitative measures for CPNs, in *Stress and Coping in Mental Health Nursing* (eds J. Carson, L. Fagin, and S. Ritter), Chapman and Hall, London.
Cartwright, S. and Cooper, C. (1997) *Managing Workplace Stress*, Sage Publications, London.
Carver, C. Scheier, M. and Weintraub, J. (1989) Assessing coping strategies: a theoretically based approach. *Journal of Personality and Social Psychology*, **56** (2), 267–83.
Cooper, C. (1986) Job distress: recent research and the emerging role of the clinical occupational psychologist. *Bulletin of the British Psychological Society*, **39**, 325–31.
Cooper, C. (1996) Stress in the workplace. *British Journal of Hospital Medicine*, **55** (9), 559–63.

Cooper, C. Sloan, J. and Williams, S. (1988) *Occupational Stress Indicator Management Guide*, NFER–Nelson, Windsor.

Cox, T. (1978) *Stress*, Macmillan, London.

Cox, T. (1993) *Stress Research and Stress Management: Putting Theory to Work*, Centre for Organizational Health and Development, University of Nottingham, Nottingham.

Cushway, D. and Tyler, P. (1996) Stress in clinical psychologists. *The International Journal of Social Psychiatry*, **42** (2), 141–9.

DCP (1995) *Professional Practice Guidelines*, Division of Clinical Psychology, British Psychological Society, Leicester.

Deary, I. Agius, R. and Sadler, A. (1996) Personality and stress in consultant psychiatrists. *The International Journal of Social Psychiatry*, **42** (2), 112–23.

Dollard, M. and Winefield, A. (1996) Managing occupational stress: a national and international perspective. *International Journal of Stress Management*, **3** (2), 69–83.

Dua, J. (1996) Development of a scale to assess occupational stress in rural general practitioners. *International Journal of Stress Management*, **3** (2), 117–28.

Eysenck, H. and Eysenck, S. (1975) *Manual for the Eysenck Personality Questionnaire*, Hodder and Stoughton, London.

Fagin, L. Carson, J. Leary, J. *et al.* (1996) Stress, coping and burnout: Findings from three research studies. *The International Journal of Social Psychiatry*, **42** (2), 102–11.

Firth-Cozens, J. (1987) Emotional distress in junior house officers. *British Medical Journal*, **295**, 533–6.

Freedy, J. and Hobfoll, S. (1994) Stress innoculation for reduction of burnout: a conservation of resources approach. *Anxiety, Stress and Coping*, **6**, 311–25.

Gibson, F. McGrath, A. and Reid, N. (1989) Occupational stress in social work. *British Journal of Social Work*, **19** (1), 1–18.

Glenister, D. (1996) Exercise and mental health: a review. *Journal of the Royal Society of Health*, February, 7–13.

Goldberg, D. and Williams, P. (1988) *A User's Guide to the General Health Questionnaire*, NFER–Nelson, Windsor.

Gordon, A. (1994) Organizational stress and stress management programmes. *International Journal of Stress Management*, **1** (4), 309–22.

Grey-Toft, P. and Anderson, J. (1981) The Nursing Stress Scale: The development of an instrument. *Journal of Behavioural Assessment*, **3**, 11–23.

Harris, P. (1989) The Nurse Stress Index. *Work and Stress*, **3** (4), 335–46.

Hipwell, A. Tyler, P. and Wilson, C. (1989) Sources of stress and dissatisfaction among nurses in four hospital environments. *British Journal of Medical Psychology*, **62**, 71–9.

Holmes, T. and Rahe, R. (1967) The Social Readjustment Rating Scale. *Journal of Psychosomatic Research*, **11**, 213–18.

Hyman, R. (1993) Evaluation of an intervention for staff in a long term facility using a retrospective pretest design. *Evaluation and the Health Professions*, **16** (2), 212–24.

Jex, S. (1991) The psychological benefits of exercise in work settings: a review. *Work and Stress*, **5** (2), 133–47.

Jones, F. Fletcher, B. and Ibbetson, K. (1991) Stresses and strains amongst social workers, demands, supports, constraints, and psychological health. *British Journal of Social Work*, **21** (5), 443–70.

Kanner, A. Coyne, J. Schaefer, C. and Lazarus, R. (1981) Comparison of two modes of stress management: daily hassles and uplifts versus major life events. *Journal of Behavioural Medicine*, **4**, 1–39.

Kerr, J. and Vlaswinkel, E. (1995) Sports participation at work: an aid to stress management. *International Journal of Stress Management*, **2** (2), 87–96.

Kobassa, S. and Puccetti, M. (1983) Personality and social resources in stress resistance. *Journal of Personality and Social Psychology*, **45** (4), 839–50.

Koeske, G. Kirk, S. and Koeske, R. (1993) Coping with work stress: which strategies work best? *Journal of Occupational and Organizational Psychology*, **66**, 319–35.

Kunkler, J. and Whittick, J. (1991) Stress management groups for nurses: practical problems and possible solutions. *Journal of Advanced Nursing*, **16**, 172–6.

Lazarus, R. (1995) Psychological stress in the workplace, in *Occupational Stress: a Handbook* (eds R. Crandall and P. Perrewe), Taylor and Francis, Washington.

Lazarus, R. and Folkman, S. (1984) *Stress, Appraisal and Coping*, Springer, New York.

Lee, S. and Crockett, M. (1994) Effect of assertiveness training on levels of stress and assertiveness experienced by nurses in Taiwan, Republic of China. *Issues in Mental Health Nursing*, **15**, 419–32.

Leiter, M. and Harvie, P. (1996) Burnout among mental health workers: A review and research agenda. *The International Journal of Social Psychiatry*, **42** (2), 90–101.

Lester, N. Nebel, L. and Baum, A. (1994) Psychophysiological and behavioural measurement of stress: applications to mental health, in *Stress and Mental Health: Contemporary Issues and Prospects for the Future* (eds W. Avison and I. Gotlib), Plenum, New York.

Long, B. and Flood, K. (1993) Coping with work stress: psychological benefits of exercise. *Work and Stress*, **7** (2), 109–19.

Martin, E. (1992) Designing stress training, in *Stress and Well Being at Work: Assessments and Interventions for Occupational Mental Health* (eds J. Quick, L. Murphy and J. Hurrell), American Psychological Association, Washington.

Maslach, C. (1993) Burnout: a multidimensional perspective, in *Professional Burnout: Recent Developments in Theory and Research* (eds W. Schaufeli, C. Maslach and T. Marek), Taylor and Francis, Washington.

Maslach, C. and Jackson, S. (1986) *Maslach Burnout Inventory*. Consulting Psychologists Press, Palo Alto.

Meichenbaum, D. (1985) *Stress Innoculation Training*, Pergamon, Elmsford, NY.

Michie, S. and Sandhu, S. (1994) Stress management for clinical medical students. *Medical Education*, **28**, 528–33.

Murphy, L. (1988) Workplace interventions for stress reduction and prevention, in *Causes, Coping and Consequences of Stress at Work* (eds C. Cooper and R. Payne), John Wiley, Chichester.

Newton, T. (1995) *Managing Stress: Emotion and Power at Work*, Sage Publications, London.

Oliver, N. and Kuipers, E. (1996) Stress and its relationship to expressed emotion in community mental health workers. *The International Journal of Social Psychiatry*, **42** (2), 150–9.

Pearlin, L. Menaghan, E. Lieberman, M. and Mullan, J. (1981) The stress process. *Journal of Health and Social Behaviour*, **22**, 337–56.

Pottage, D. and Huxley, P. (1996) Stress and mental health social work: a developmental perspective. *The International Journal of Social Psychiatry*, **42** (2), 124–31.

Reynolds, S. and Briner, R. (1994) Stress management at work: with whom, for whom, and to what ends? *British Journal of Guidance and Counselling*, **22** (1), 75–89.

Richardsen, A. and Burke, R. (1995) Models of burnout: implications for interventions. *International Journal of Stress Management*, **2** (1), 31–43.

Roger, D. and Hudson, C. (1995) The role of emotion control and emotional rumination in stress management training. *International Journal of Stress Management*, **2** (3), 119–32.

Rosch, P. (1994) Stress management training: Why all the fuss?' *International Journal of Stress Management*, **1** (3), 217–22.

Ross, R. and Altmaier, E. (1994) *Intervention in Occupational Stress*, Sage Publications, London.

Sauter, S. Murphy, L. and Hurrell, J. (1990) Prevention of work related psychological disorders: a national strategy proposed by the National Institute for Occupational Safety and Health (NIOSH). *American Psychologist*, **45**, 146–58.

Schaufeli, W. Enzman, D. and Girault, N. (1993) Measurement of burnout: A review, in *Professional Burnout: Recent Developments in Theory and Research* (eds W. Schaufeli, C. Maslach and T. Marek), Taylor and Francis, Washington.

Snow, D. and Kline, M. (1995) Preventive interventions in the workplace to reduce negative psychiatric consequences of work and family stress, in *Does Stress Cause Psychiatric Illness?* (ed. C. Mazure), American Psychiatric Press, Washington.

Sweeney, G. and Nichols, K. (1996) Stress experiences of occupational therapists in mental health practice arenas: a review of the literature. *The International Journal of Social Psychiatry*, **42** (2), 132–40.

Sweeney, G. Nichols, K. and Kline, P. (1991) Factors contributing to work related stress in occupational therapists: results from a pilot study. *British Journal of Occupational Therapy*, **54** (8), 284–8.

Sweeney, G. Nichols, K. and Cormack, M. (1993) Job stress in occupational therapy: coping strategies, stress management techniques, and recommendations for change. *British Journal of Occupational Therapy*, **56** (4), 140–5.

Turner, R. and Roszell, P. (1994) Psychosocial resources and the stress process, in *Stress and Mental Health: Contemporary Issues and Prospects for the Future* (eds W. Avison, and L. Gotlib), Plenum, New York.

Walsh, S. Nichols, K. and Cormack, M. (1991) Self care and clinical psychologists: a threatening obligation? *Clinical Psychology Forum*, **37**, 5–7.

Weiss, D. Dawis, R. England, G. and Lofquist, L. (1977) *Minnesota Satisfaction Questionnaire: Short Form*, University of Minnesota, Minnesota.

Stressed staff: implications for staff selection | 13

Ben Thomas

INTRODUCTION

The selection of the right staff for the job is a key component of all successful organisations. Nowhere is this more important than in the area of health care, where the recruitment of the best staff is necessary for the attainment of a high quality service. The implications of poor selection are well known. On the one hand, selecting people without the right skills, ability, and aptitude may well result in dramatic consequences for the organization in terms of poor performance, high levels of sickness, and low morale. Promotion above a person's level of competence can also have a devastating effect on that individual. People who are ill-equipped to carry out the job for which they have been appointed will undoubtedly suffer anxiety and stress. These problems are often compounded when individuals are not able to share their doubts, uncertainties, and fears, and they are left unsupported and without guidance for the future. On the other hand, selecting people who are overqualified for the job may also result in the individual becoming bored, frustrated, and disillusioned, particularly if the organization is unable to accommodate people reaching their potential through career development.

The NHS is labour intensive and like other public services views itself as a fair and model employer (Farnham, 1993). Securing an adequately skilled work force is a major target for NHS Trusts. Government policy over the past few years has been to try and increase employee productivity. In the main this was expected to occur through local determination of pay and conditions. As well as rewarding good performance, local pay determination was supposed to enable Trusts to respond to local labour market conditions.

In addition to local pay determination the Government's reforms have introduced a range of initiatives related to the NHS work force, including skill mix reviews, equal opportunities, employee relations, performance appraisal, health care workers, and extensive recruitment and retention campaigns. These new developments all seek to bring about attitudinal and cultural changes in the NHS. The value placed on an effective work force is underpinned by the understanding that it is crucial to select the right person for the job.

DISCRIMINATION

The selection of staff begins with the implementation of a fair and open recruitment process. In fact it is unlawful to discriminate against people during any stage of the recruitment and selection process because of their gender, race, nationality, ethnic origins or because they are married. Over the past few years the NHS has made significant strides to establish recruitment and selection procedures based on non-discriminatory work-related criteria. However, recent research suggests that there still exist large gaps between equal opportunity policies and actual practice in the workplace. For example, despite approximately 8 per cent of NHS nursing and midwifery staff being from ethnic minority groups racial inequality remains a significant problem. Recent research by Beishon, Virdee and Hagell (1995) suggests that ethnic minority nurses, particularly black nurses, had not advanced as far up the grading structure as their white colleagues, even after controlling for other career factors such as qualifications and length of time in the profession.

The importance of staff selection has been heightened by the adverse publicity recently given to matters racial and sexual discrimination, malpractice, and ill-treatment of patients – for example, the Allitt Inquiry (HMSO, 1994) into the circumstances surrounding the murder of four children and the injuring of nine others in the children's ward of Grantham and Kesteven Hospital in 1991. Among a number of recommendations, the need for formal health screening was highlighted. Also recommended was the availability to occupational health departments of any records of absence through sickness. The report emphasized that no candidate for nursing with evidence of major personality disorder should be employed.

Beverly Allitt is described as having a malevolent, deranged criminal mind; however, her case serves to raise questions about the selection of health service staff with a history of mental illness or illnesses related to stress. Whereas it is accepted practice for health care professionals to be properly screened, particularly those wishing to work with vulnerable groups, screening methods and employment practices must be anti-discriminatory. Mental health service users have fought long and hard to work in partnership with mental health professionals. Many Trusts have set up advisory and consultation systems so that service users are able to contribute to service planning and delivery. Pathfinder Mental Health Services NHS Trust in south London has taken the initiative of actively seeking to recruit nurses and other clinical staff with mental health problems. The Trust is aiming for one in ten of its employees to be users or ex-users of mental health services. The recent repeal of the Disabled Persons (Employment) Act 1944 by the Disability Act 1995 means that discrimination against people with disabilities is now on a similar footing with sex or racial discrimination. It is unlawful for employers to treat a person less favourably due to disability and an employer is obliged to make reasonable changes within the organization to prevent disadvantage occurring, for example changing working hours.

WORK-FORCE PLANNING

As the shortage of health service staff increases, selecting the right people with the necessary skills for each job is a daunting task for many organizations. National work-force planning in the NHS has been a hit-and-miss exercise. As a result there are shortages in most of the clinical professions, including medicine, nursing, psychology, and speech therapy. The Royal College of Nursing reports that in 1996 there were 13,000 trainee nurses compared with 37,000 in 1983. There are particular shortages in the specialities. For example there is an increasing shortage of mental health nurses. Recently the shortage of anaesthetists has received widespread publicity. There is a chronic shortage of paediatric nurses and according to the Audit Commission only 17 per cent of Trusts are meeting RCN staffing requirements. There is an increasing turnover and wastage of nurses generally. Despite these shortages and the growing demand on nurses to work additional hours, the Institute of Employment Studies (1995) has reported nurses' perceptions of growing job insecurity and deteriorating career prospects.

A recent survey of nurse managers conducted by the *Health Service Journal* painted a similar picture (Dix, 1996). Many nurse managers are demoralized about their future prospects and believe that nursing management is a threatened profession. They reported feeling insecure in their jobs, overworked, and inadequately supported. A fifth of those who responded felt so disillusioned that they were thinking of leaving the NHS.

According to the National Association of Health Authorities and Trusts (NAHAT, 1996) 80 per cent of Trusts are experiencing difficulty recruiting consultants. Either no one applies for advertised vacancies, too few apply, or the applicants are not suitable for the job. NAHAT found that high drop-out rates among consultants and junior doctors was a significant cause of current recruitment problems.

Against this background of stress, low morale, and uncertainty, where demand seems to be outstripping supply, great care must be taken in selecting the right person for each job. Most selection processes are constructed around tried and tested methods. These include advertising the job, receiving applications, shortlisting, interviewing, taking up references, interviewing again, and making an appointment. Recently, these have been supplemented by other, newer techniques.

SELECTION PROCEDURES

Selection is defined as the process of assessing applicants and choosing whom to employ. Traditional methods of selecting staff are geared towards finding someone who can do the job. For many years in the NHS once a post became vacant it was more or less automatically refilled, often without any thought to the necessity or appropriateness of that role. With moves towards a businesslike environment, increased efficiency, rapid developments in technologies, continual restructuring, and reforms in working arrangements, staff often find themselves taking on responsibilities different to those they expected. Although it is more commonplace for an existing vacancy to be reappraised and the nature of the job re-examined, this approach still sees recruitment from only the organization's perspective. A more enlightened approach not only takes into consideration the nature of the job and the skills, qualifications, experience, and personal qualities necessary to undertake that role, but also considers recruitment from the applicant's perspective. The importance of the candidate's ability to fit into the organization is acknowledged. Many organizations also appreciate the stress that newcomers will experience and seek to minimize this whenever possible.

Job descriptions

In health care, job descriptions and personal specifications are usually drawn up by senior clinical staff in collaboration with the personnel or human resources department. Importance is accorded to the job title as this should reflect a true picture of what is expected of the post holder. This is particularly relevant in nursing because of the wide variety of work within the profession. In recent years there has been a proliferation of nursing titles, including primary nurse, staff nurse, charge nurse, practice nurse, ward manager, lecturer/practitioner, specialist practitioner, practice development nurse, clinical nurse specialist, advanced practitioner. This array of titles is often confusing to patients, relatives, and other staff.

Most job descriptions consist of a number of key tasks or main objectives. Often included in the description are organizational structures, communication channels, and lines of accountability. Personal specifications are usually divided into essential and desirable criteria. Essential criteria include professional and educational qualifications, level of experience required (including special experience), personal qualities (such as problem-solving ability), interpersonal skills, the need to communicate verbally and in writing. Desirable criteria may include the ability to train and teach people, computing skills, and the ability to drive and the right to hold a driving licence.

Recruitment

The purpose of recruitment is to attract a number of suitable applicants to apply for the job in question. In order to do so it is necessary to bring to the attention of the target audience that a vacancy exists. This can be done in a number of ways, including targeting internal candidates through newsletters, noticeboards, memos, e-mail circulars, and direct approaches. External candidates can be targeted through advertising, using media such as newspapers, radio and television, professional journals, job fairs, posters, and open days.

Advertising is still regarded as the most effective way of reaching a wide selection of potential candidates. A noticeable change has occurred in advertising for health care professionals. The shortage of suitably qualified staff has led to greater competition, which in turn has resulted in organizations paying particular attention to the design of their advertisements. Advertisements are often large and designed to catch the eye of potential candidates. For example some organizations use colour, a logo, or a gimmick designed to attract candidates. Figure 13.1 shows a recruitment questionnaire from the Bethlem and Maudsley NHS Trust, which offered a prize draw of £250. Many organizations highlight the attractive opportunities and facilities that exist. In fact many organizations now offer added incentives to attract staff, including accommodation, crèche facilities, sporting opportunities, and professional development and training. However, it is important to give potential applicants as realistic a picture as possible of the organization; otherwise expectations will be raised and disappointment will ensue which may ultimately result in high staff turnover.

Attention needs to be given to the timing of an advert, as well as to choosing the right medium for it. Most people do not bother to advertise around bank holidays or long summer holidays. Many nursing posts are often coordinated and advertised together. However, the advantages and disadvantages of a decision to delay advertising should be carefully considered, as it may well lose potential candidates and demotivate existing staff.

Applications

Most organizations have their own application forms. These can be useful in that they enable the provision of standard information. However, they usually only provide a minimal amount of data; so whenever possible candidates should be given the opportunity to provide a curriculum vitae. It is good practice to inform each applicant that their application has been received and is being considered. It is important that the whole interviewing team is involved in drawing up the shortlist for interview and that everyone works from the set criteria.

Shortlisting

Shortlisting should be carried out systematically, relying on the essential and desirable criteria previously decided. Most organizations produce a grid of the selection criteria for this purpose, eliminating anyone who does not meet the essential criteria. Shortlisting is problematic when there are either too many applicants or not enough. The former calls for the very rigorous application of essential criteria

We need mental health nurses to
Tell us the Truth

The Maudsley is committed to recruiting and retaining the best nurses. Our aim is to attract qualified nurses to work for us, so that we can provide a high quality, accessible and appropriate clinical service to all our patients.

Listening to you is the first step in helping us to set the agenda for future recruitment and retention strategies. Completing and returning this questionnaire is your opportunity to tell us what you want.

To thank you for your time, we will be entering all completed questionnaires in a draw with a £250 prize. The draw will be held on 4 October 1995 and the winner will be notified by 11 October 1995.

Please return your completed questionnaire to Pamela Tibbles, Head of Nursing Practice, FREEPOST (licence no. SE5477). The Bethlem and Maudsley NHS Trust, Monks Orchard Road, Beckenham, Kent BR3 3BX.

Q If you were looking for a new post in nursing, what grade would you be looking for?
A ....
   ....

Q Which areas of Psychiatry would you be interested in working in?
A ....
   ....

Q What would be your preferred days/hours of work?
A ....
   ....

Q If you are not currently nursing, would you be interested in undertaking a 'Return to Practice' course?
A YES ○   NO ○

   If yes is this in order to regain UKCC registration?
   YES ○   NO ○

Q What sort of professional development would you be looking for?
A ....
   ....

Q Please indicate which of the facilities below would attract you to come and work for the Trust in London?
A ○ Subsidised day nursery
   ○ Financial help with childcare
   ○ After-school and holiday club
   ○ Social club
   ○ Healthcare facilities
   ○ Sports facilities
   ○ Shopping facilities
   ○ Accommodation
      ○ Family
      ○ Single
      ○ Long-term
      ○ Short-term
   ○ Practical help with finding accommodation
   ○ Other ....

Do you have any further comments?
....
....
....

£250 prize draw The questionnaire is anonymous, but if you would like your name to be entered in the draw, please complete this section, which will be detached from the questionnaire on receipt.

NAME:...
TELEPHONE NUMBER:...
The prize has kindly been donated from charitable funds.

THE MAUDSLEY
Advancing mental health care

Figure 13.1 Recruitment questionnaire from the Bethlem and Maudsley NHS Trust.

and the latter an analysis of the selection criteria and the marketing and advertising strategy. It is important that a poor response does not force people into short-listing unsuitable candidates.

Informal visits

Informal visits should provide the candidate with an opportunity to gain some insight into the working environment and the people with whom they will have contact. Informal visits should be relaxed, with as much time as possible given to the candidate to ask questions. It is inevitable that impressions of the candidate's suitability for the post will be formed at informal visits, but they should not be used as an additional interview.

Interviews

For the most part, employers still regard interviews as the traditional method of staff selection. However, the style and content of interviews vary considerably. Many interviewers do not like having to think up questions for themselves. One response to creating a more thorough and fair system has been the introduction of behaviourally based or targeted interviews. These are based on the assumption that past performance is the best indicator of future performance. Candidates are asked a list of predetermined questions which are geared to establishing whether the candidate can provide behavioural evidence as proof of each competency. Such a technique has received a mixed reception, particularly in the USA where this type of interviewing was accepted earlier than in the UK. In addition there are a number of other approaches that are now more commonly adopted, including formal presentations and psychological assessment.

Interviewing

Interviews are still the most commonly used of all selection methods. Despite their being universally used, most people find them a harrowing experience. As far as possible in the NHS, the employer should do their best to put people at their ease. It is important for all concerned that the candidates are able to function and present themselves as best they can and that the interviewing team is seen as representing the value system of the organization. Yet, time and time again we hear of employers whose idea of an interview is to give people a tough time. In fact many interviews these days are known as 'stress interviews' since they are specifically designed to throw people off balance. However, such a process often leaves people humiliated and traumatized, as described by Kate Herbert (1996). There are some basic principles that employers should follow. These include being organized before the interviews, choosing a suitable venue where there will be no interruptions, providing a comfortable waiting area, supplying refreshments, starting on time, and informing the candidate how long the interview is likely to last.

Although it is important for interviewers to be representative of the major stakeholders the interview panel should be kept as small as possible.

Selecting appropriate questions is often difficult. However, they should be unambiguous and as fair as possible. Asking candidates about their achievements in their last or present job can bring to light their skills and motivation. Questions about their strengths, weaknesses, and training needs will provide information about their competencies and abilities, including the ability to grow in the job.

To obain evidence of an applicant's suitability requires questioning skills from the interviewer. Direct questions are useful for extracting or clarifying information, while probing questions are useful for finding out more information. For example, asking a candidate to describe a situation where they had conflict with another individual and how they dealt with it may provide some valuable insight into leadership and dealing with conflict. Hypothetical questions are useful for examining how people might react in certain circumstances. Most interview panels meet beforehand and agree an interviewing format, including which members of the panel will cover the different aspects of the job.

In their tips for doing well at job interviews, London University Careers Service suggest that employers want to know three things and will ask a variety of questions to elicit the information: Can the person do the job? Will the person do the job? Will the person fit in? Their other tips include:

- Know the job. The candidate should reread the job description and think about what evidence they can present that will show that they already have the appropriate skills.
- Know the organization. The candidate should find out what they can (for instance, information from the annual report) and they should also make sure they know the location, time, and date of the interview.
- Try to relax. The candidate should breathe slowly and deeply before going into the interview.
- Don't give yes or no answers. The candidate should speak slowly and clearly, giving answers that volunteer relevant information about themselves. They should always answer the question without going off at a tangent.
- Be truthful, but positive. Even if the candidate is talking about a weakness or failure, they should talk about how they overcame it or what they learned.
- Seek clarification. If a person does not understand a question they should say so; they may, but not too often, ask for a little time to think.
- The candidate should realize that they may be dealing with a trained and organized professional interviewer – or with someone who simply bases their decisions on a gut reaction, is likely to be disorganised, may ask closed yes/no questions and may themselves talk far too much. The candidate should be prepared to spot the difference between the two and respond positively to help the process in their favour.
- Deadly traps the person should avoid include failing to listen to the questions, answering a question that was not asked, providing superfluous information, and attempting to conduct their interview without adequate preparation.

Presentations

Formal presentations have become very popular over the past few years as an additional method of assessing candidates to see if they can convey information in a concise, understandable, and well thought out style. Presentations also provide material from which to ask the candidates questions later in the interview. Although the time allocated to presentations may differ, it is usually in the region of ten to twenty minutes. All candidates are given the same question to address and they are judged not only on the relevance of their presentation and their grasp of the important issues but also on style and ability. Particular attention is paid to how the candidate engages the listener, manages their own anxiety, and handles questions. Formal presentations provide a focus for the candidates in preparing for the interview; they also provide candidates with an opportunity to impart their knowledge in a structured form and demonstrate their ability to communicate.

Psychological assessment

Psychological assessment is aimed at providing an evaluation of a candidate's abilities. Billsberry (1996) suggests that personality, literacy, numeracy, and intelligence tests are now used by approximately half the organizations in Britain for some of their vacancies. Billsbury provides a bar chart which shows the frequency of the use of selection techniques by organizations in the UK. Psychological assessments are used as an aid to help make professional judgements about candidates and are valuable in selecting the person who would best fit a particular job. In the NHS they have usually been confined to senior management selection. However, they can be used at any level of job selection in assessing potential, in trying to find the best person to fit a particular job, or where performance problems need to be explored. They are thought to be a practical means of obtaining information that could otherwise be time consuming to collect. Psychological tests are only of value if they are used for the purpose for which they were designed and are employed in the context of other information about a person. Fletcher (1996) argues that if the job requirements are clearly defined then it is better to use role-specific personality questionnaires that are tailored to the purpose.

References

The purpose of references is to verify what the applicant has disclosed on their application form and during the interview. It is common practice for employers to seek at least two references from most applicants. One is expected from the current or last employer and one from a previous employer, college, or university. As a minimum the reference should contain details about the referee's professional relationship with the candidate, length of employment, ability, reliability, qualities and skills, and sickness and absenteeism record. These details are meant to aid prospective employers confirm information already provided by the applicant and make a prediction about their future performance (Cooper and Robertson, 1995).

Feedback and counselling

If individuals are to learn from their interview experience, feedback is crucial. Such feedback may also involve counselling and career guidance. Feedback will help support people, review their progress, and identify their strengths and weaknesses. Counselling may also help support individuals who have been unsuccessful in their application by allowing them to express their feelings of disappointment, anger, or frustration and providing opportunity to talk through future plans. Career guidance can help define an individual's skills and competencies and clarify their aims for the future. This will help people take responsibility for their own career development.

Education, training, and development

The importance of responding to the needs of staff is highlighted by David Sines in Chapter 7. This includes providing appropriate opportunities for continuing education and training for staff. It is vital for people to keep up to date, to maintain and enhance their skills, to practise safely, and to feel confident about their work. Providing staff with individual development and training opportunities is a means of valuing staff. Most people have drives towards personal growth and development if provided with an environment that is supportive and encouraging. This means not only providing training on the job to achieve better performance but also being interested in the wider development of the individual.

CONCLUSION

With the increasing shortage of qualified NHS staff it is likely that recruitment will become much more aggressive and competitive. The shortage of staff requires urgent attention and may require a national overview of recruitment needs since the future of the health service depends on having a capable and flexible work force. Selecting the right staff is vital to the future success of the NHS, using appropriate methods will cut down turnover and attract those people who are going to make a difference to the services we provide. Selection involves judgement and choice. It is more important than ever that we choose the right person for the job and for the organization, thereby increasing job satisfaction and reducing work related stress.

From an individual's perspective the frequent changes in organizational structures within the current health service have often meant fewer promotional opportunities, loss of job security, and changing values. This has resulted in many professionals seeking opportunities for which they are either not suited or not yet ready. The preoccupation with the management function has led many good clinical professionals to take on management roles and responsibilities. While the non-clinical aspects of the NHS continue to grow, many of those clinicians who have taken on a managerial role find it unfulfilling and stressful and want to return to a clinical focus. The need for a flexible work force and the loss of upward progression has resulted in lateral moves and role adaptation. Again there are those who find adaptation easy and those who find the transition uncomfortable and stressful.

The health service and its employees have to face up to the need to make staff selection as effective as possible. The cost of selecting the right person for the job can be significant but the benefits far outweigh the detrimental effects of poor selection, which can often result in a tragic situation for both the organization and the individual.

REFERENCES

Beishon, S., Virdee, S. and Hagell, A. (1995) *Nursing in a Multi-Ethnic NHS*, Policy Studies Institute, London.

Billsberry, J. (1996) *Finding and Keeping the Right People: How to Recruit Motivated Employees*, Pitman Publishing, London.

Cooper, D. and Robertson, I.T. (1995) *The Psychology of Personnel Selection*, Routledge, London.

Dix (1996) Tales by the Nurses Grim. *Health Service Journal*, **106** (5500), 38–9.

Farnham, D. (1993) Human resources management and employer relations, in *Managing The New Public Services* (eds D. Farnham and S. Horton), Macmillan, London.

Fletcher, C. (1996) When focusing on the specifics is more valid. *People Management*, **2** (10), 47.

Herbert, K. (1996) *The Guardian*, 29 June.

HMSO (1994) The Allitt Inquiry: Independent inquiry relating to deaths and injuries on the children's ward at Grantham and Kesteven Hospital during the period February to April 1991. HMSO, London.

The Institute of Employment Studies (1995) *Recruiting, Retaining and Rewarding Qualified Nurses in 1995*, Brighton.

NAHAT (1996) Is there a doctor in the house? *Health Director*, **25**, 10–11.

14

Personal experiences of stress at work

Patrick Hopkinson, Sally Hardy and Jerome Carson

A NEST OF VIPERS

Whenever personal experiences of stress caused by work-related problems rears its head, it is met with a varied response from work colleagues. Some are sympathetic, others dismissive, but overall comes the sense of 'we'd rather not know'. Denying that caring for others as a profession has a deterimental side effect on one's mental health is both ridiculous and ignorant. Harsh words perhaps, but as the suicide numbers mount within the health care professional group, evidence suggests that things cannot be ignored without drastic consequences.

Reseach into the field of stress at work for health professionals remains sparse. This can be put down to problems with the highly subjective nature of stress, but can also be seen as opening a nest of vipers. The sample population are renowned for being poor recipients of health care themselves, avoiding contact with services, and maintaining a belief that it should not happen to them as professional carers. Obtaining contact with health professionals who suffer mental health problems is difficult and getting them to discuss their problems openly is shrouded with litigation risks. All of this is a means of safeguarding the profession and oneself. Avoiding the reality helps one to deny those all too familiar feelings of fear, guilt, rage, and helplessness. Yet research is being carried out and the most appropriate methods are being tried and tested. There is still so much to be learnt from people's personal experiences that can help others and that offers a basis of knowledge that will help those in the caring professions to continue to care to the best of their abilities.

Our interest in occupational stress comes from varied routes. All three of us can identify times in our careers when we felt like giving it all up for a stress-free existence, but the rewards and gains outweighed the upheaval of starting all over again. Two of us (JC and SH) were interviewed for a radio programme on health care worker stress. We discussed the research we were involved in and our personal experiences. At the end of the taped interview the interviewer admitted to having become interested in mental health issues after a close relative had tragically taken their life. Whatever it takes to get people more aware and interested in mental health issues is as diverse and extreme as can be expected. This chapter covers some of the diverse and unexpected aspects of personal experiences of stress and tries to help us make sense of them.

This chapter divides into three sections. First we present three case studies, then some of the research methods that can be applied to this sort of information, and finally a section on how to go about doing a research project using the techniques described. The chapter is concerned with exploring the meaning of statements people make about the stress they experience. It also considers how the analysis of these statements can be used to add a further dimension to the study of occupational stress. To begin, there is a brief summary of the major differences between the use of traditionally valid quantitative (usually statistical) analyses of stress-causing factors and the use of qualitative methods to deal with the data without the necessity of turning it into numerical form. Following this, advice is given on how to carry out a qualitative research and analysis project, with an example taken from a research study on the psychological effect on hospital nurses caring for the suicidal patient.

CASE EXAMPLE 1

'Can you tell me about a recent event at work that you found particularly stressful?'

> I decided to visit a client after 5 p.m. on a Friday, on my way home. I thought it would be a simple visit; just pop in to see him for a short while and then head off for the weekend. He let me in and said that he had something to show me. I remember feeling a little surprised about this but also genuinely interested to find out what it was. He had been feeling very depressed recently and I was quite pleased to find that he was at least beginning to show some interest in something. I said, 'Okay,' and he turned around, opened a drawer, and reached into it. He then turned to face me and stretched out his hand. He was holding a gun!
>
> I didn't know what to do. I stood frozen to the spot for what seemed like ages. Finally for a reason I still can't work out, I said, 'Please, give me the gun.' I remember feeling really silly. I mean, there he was, standing in front of me with a gun and I was asking him to give it me. It was like a film, but this was real. I can't really recall feeling so scared!
>
> He said, 'It's not loaded,' and then put the gun back in the drawer. My heart was pounding but I kept thinking, 'I've got to act professionally; I can't show I'm frightened; I'm the one who's meant to be calm. What will he do if he sees that I'm panicking?'

I didn't know whether to stay or make my excuses and leave. We don't have an out of hours on-call system and I was really worried about how he would be over the weekend. I remember realizing that I hadn't told anyone where I was going! I felt totally alone. I could have been killed and no one else would have known.

It was later on at home that the full extent dawned on me. I was traumatized. I couldn't sit still and felt really agitated. I suppose I had been in shock when it happened and hadn't had time to think about it. Suddenly I felt tears welling up and I burst out crying. All that stress came to the surface and I couldn't control it. I felt really desperate. I was a grown man who had seen disturbing and unpleasant things when I had worked in hospitals. I suppose then I had other people to share the experience with and at least I wasn't on my own when things happened. Now I realized how important that had been for me. I also kept thinking about, I suppose, practical things, like: Should I contact the police? What was I going to do?'

CASE EXAMPLE 2

'How do you feel about your present situation at work?'

It was the last thing I had expected (being made redundant). Of course, I'm more used to it now but then, well, then I was building my career, getting better-paid positions, climbing up the ladder. Actually, I'd just read a book on management which had a chapter on organizational decline in it. Quite ironic.

When I heard that I was 'surplus to requirements', so to speak, I went through the same process of bereavement the book had mentioned. At first, I couldn't believe it. I thought, well, we'll see, I bet in a few weeks it'll be all right; it won't actually happen.

One thing that really got at me was that the night before I heard about all this, we were planning a pretty expensive holiday. We were going to book it the day after and it would be something to look forward to. When I found out about redundancy, that stopped those plans, I can tell you! It felt so unfair. I couldn't arrange anything over the next few months. It was like the whole year was being affected and I couldn't do anything to stop it. I suppose I discovered how important work was in making sense of life and giving it some order. Finding out in February that I would be without work in April meant that a whole chunk of the year was written off. I had to start finding a new job.

Then I got to thinking, hang on, how am I supposed to find a job quite as convenient for me as this one? I lived within walking distance, got 30 days holiday a year, a contracted 35 hour week, a decent pension scheme … I'd never taken as much interest in terms and conditions before! I was pretty angry, argued with my partner over really petty things, and then used to sit in the spare room feeling utterly motivationless and despondent. At other times, I'd go through a job-seeking frenzy. I'd virtually devour the newspaper looking for anything I could do. I didn't really care what it was. There were other things too, like a really strange feeling of calm sometimes. I used to just stop what I was doing and just sit there not actually feeling anything.

Thinking about it now, the disruption really upset me. All the things I'd planned were now meaningless. I'd been thinking about buying a new car – couldn't even contemplate that now. I had to really watch how much money I was spending, I started to work out exactly how much a month I needed to survive. You don't get your mortgage paid when you're redundant. I felt really close to the edge. I didn't want to look over it. You hear about all those people who used to work in the City who were laid off and the troubles they had. I'd never even imagined that I would be in a similar position.

Working out my notice period has been really difficult. It's been hard to be motivated when I know I'll not be there any more in a few weeks. The stress I feel from doing this is really intense and it dominates me. I'm not going to get a large redundancy package, I've got a few interviews to go through. My mind's not on the job. I think about me and what I am going to do. There's a definite sense of unreality about the whole situation. Now I suppose I'm resigned to it. I'm still not happy, still get despondent, and still get angry. Life's like that, isn't it?

CASE EXAMPLE 3

'What areas in your work do you find stressful?'

There's never enough time to fit everything in. I'm always finding that I take work home with me, every evening and also at weekends. I may not always do it, but I've got it there with me. Actually, when I do take work home with me and I plan to do it, I'll say to myself, 'No, I'll do it in an hour; I'll watch TV now'. After that hour, I'll put it off a bit more. Finally, I think, well it's too late now, I need to go to bed to be any good tomorrow. But, I've spent all evening thinking about it – I might as well have done it.

Often on a Monday morning in the shower, I'll think about all the things I'll have to do when I get to work. I almost get a sense of doom! There are times at work when I'm feeling particularly pressured that I actually try to avoid people. That's really hard because my job involves meeting with and talking to people all the time.

Sometimes I think about getting out of my job altogether and doing something less stressful. I know that I won't but it's a way of coping – to dream about an easier life. Maybe I'm an escapist.

What are my main causes of stress? Well, one thing is liaison. As I said before, sometimes when I have a lot to do it's actually just one more thing too many to actually pick up the phone and make that call. I either have several other things to do or I think, no, I'll call them tomorrow. Thinking about it, I'm always worried that when I do liaise it'll mean more work for me! It doesn't work as a way of sharing a problem all the time. Anyway, when I do phone, they're often not there so I leave a message.

I find it hard to separate my work from my home. Like I said, I'll take work home with me and even if I don't do it, I'm thinking about it. I'll spend some evenings just worrying and in fact not do anything. That really gets on my husband's nerves sometimes and that makes me feel unhappy. That's a cause of stress.

Another thing is the unpredictability of my work. I never know what I'll meet next. It's impossible to prepare for everything and I'm always expecting to hear something which will mean I have to change my plans for the rest of the week. I can't go home and then expect to come back into the office the next day to pick things up how I left them. It's the whole thing about events happening which I have absolutely no control over. That's the essence of stress for me.

Believe it or not, I find going on holiday stressful. I spend more time at work making sure everything is sorted and then maybe four days before coming back I'm thinking about what might have happened while I've been away. All the work I do before taking leave is ridiculous, passing things on to other people, making sure things won't get lost while I'm away – but they do all the same, running around arranging the meetings and the visits that have to happen before I go. You know, it would be easier if I didn't bother with holidays. All the liaison and coordination require so much time.

QUALITY OR QUANTITY?

Research methodologies are divided between two dichotomous poles (Henwood and Pidgeon, 1995; Henwood and Pidgeon, 1992). Quantitative methods employ rigorous controls in order to ensure that their results have high validity and reliability. In order to do this, laboratory studies are favoured in which the possible variables present can be controlled and manipulated. The data produced are then subjected to statistical analysis to assess whether any significant effects have been identified. This necessitates the use of experimental procedures that elicit information that is readily quantifiable. In turn, this leads to a requirement to choose areas of research that can be easily treated in this way.

Qualitative methods, however, do not necessarily demand such tight experimental controls (Miles and Huberman, 1992). They often use data collected in the field, by using interviews and observations that attempt to capture the richness of their subject matter and the complexity of real-life events (Orford, 1995).

Qualitative analysis utilizes the creativity of the researcher to identify the context and the meaning of the data (Henwood and Pigeon, 1992). It is concerned with presenting a recognizable, accurate depiction of the participants' viewpoint (Wiseman, 1978) and the language they use.

Despite this, qualitative methods do not ignore the importance of reliability and validity and can employ rigorous techniques to ensure the accuracy of their data and analysis (Miles and Huberman, 1992). Harper (1994) quotes Good and Watts' (1989) emphasis that quantitative methods are 'by no means the only way to rigour'.

What can be gained from the use of qualitative methods in the field of occupational stress research? Orford (1995) has argued that qualitative approaches concentrate on the viewpoint of the 'insider'. They explore the significance and attempt to elucidate the meaning of experiences (Banister et al., 1994). This is in opposition to the concern of quantitative research with deriving objective assessments of events from which theories can be developed.

Stress is a fundamentally subjective experience. Its causes are complex and its occurrence and effects unpredictable, yet it is a term used by a great many people to describe a phenomenon that impacts upon their lives. A qualitative approach to stress research could present the variety of personal definitions and ways of talking about stress derived by those who experience it. It could not be argued that these would be definitive, since they would be essentially personal, but they would possess an 'undeniability' (Miles and Huberman, 1992) lacking in more formally developed definitions. Qualitative methods provide a means of preserving and maintaining the impact of the data (Hopkinson et al., 1995). As an illustration, in a recent study into community psychiatric nurses' experiences of stress, one participant described their feelings about stress in their work in the following way: 'It's the demands or needs that we cannot respond to. It feels like painting on a large canvas with a small brush. There is a huge waiting list, so much could be done if resources were there. ...' (Carson et al., 1994). Arguably statements such as this have greater social meaning than academic definitions.

THE QUALITATIVE RESEARCH APPROACH

Given that qualitative methods provide a legitimate and productive approach towards the study of occupational stress, how are data in the form of verbal statements handled? The following description provides a basic conceptualization of how personal experiences of stress can be analysed. For further information and advice on this process, there are a number of highly useful resources available (e.g. Miles and Huberman, 1992; Banister et al., 1994; Silverman, 1994). Whilst there are a wide variety of qualitative methods, including grounded theory (Glaser and Strauss, 1967), discourse analysis (Harper, 1994), and verbal protocol analysis (Green, 1995), there are certain fundamental approaches to research that are shared between them.

GETTING STARTED

The initial step is the formulation of a research question or a hypothesis. This can be fairly loosely formulated but is necessary in order to guide the research and to allow data collection to be a more precise process. The greatest risk in any qualitative study is to collect too much data, which then proves too large, too complex, and too nebulous to analyse effectively (Miles and Huberman, 1992). Whilst it can be persuasively argued that specifying limits restricts the freedom offered by qualitative methods, pragmatic considerations must inevitably dictate some aspects of the research endeavour if the study is to be successful.

A research question might be, 'How do mental health workers describe stress?' or, 'Do workers who have been taught stress-coping methods talk about stress in a different way to their colleagues who have not?'

What is important to bear in mind is that the purpose of the study does not have to be the discovery of universal laws which can be extrapolated from the individual participants to all people in a similar situation (Orford, 1995). Silverman (1994) argues that an authentic account of an individual's experience is more important than a replicable, reliable measure using a number of subjects. Consequently, it is possible to set out to analyse very specific events and situations which in essence are not shared with others. However, research that offers an insight into more general events is equally possible using qualitative methods.

This leads to the decision about the number of participants. It is quite possible to conduct a qualitative study using information gathered from just one person. This idiopathic approach could produce a very rich and hopefully accurate depiction of how an individual describes their experiences, beliefs, ideas, and actions in relation to the topic under investigation. However, it must be acknowledged that this would not provide results that are easily applicable to other individuals. If this is an aim of the research then a larger number of participants is required.

It is possible to gather data from a large number of people who have a unifying characteristic, such as their job, but who otherwise could not be considered to be similar. This would make it possible not only to present the shared experiences they may have, but also to bring out the differences. Doing this could then lead to a further consideration of the factors involved in causing these similarities and idiosyncracies.

Thought must then be given to the way in which the study is to be conducted and the method used for eliciting and recording data. Since the information required to answer the research question is verbal, a means of eliciting this is necessary. Interviews are a standard method. A major issue is choosing the degree of structure to be used.

Unstructured interviews probably allow a more flexible approach in which the participant can exert their own control of the situation and consequently these are less coercive than structured methods. Naturally, a structured interview will gather more precise information and less that is not strictly relevant to the research. Deciding which is more appropriate is a matter of weighing up a number of factors including the time available for each interview, the amount of data which can be effectively handled, and the importance given to the gathering of information that might serve to add context rather than content. Open-ended questions are clearly useful, as is allowing the participant to add topics of discussion to the interview which they feel are appropriate to the purpose of the study. This can be achieved quite simply by asking them whether there is anything else they wish to say. Thus it is essential to acknowledge that the interviewee is in no way blind to the study and that in fact they are an active part of it.

Data-recording methods basically consist of hand-written accounts made during the interview or of tape-recorded transcriptions. The choice between these is often governed by the availability of recording equipment and of a suitable interview location. Tape recording offers definite advantages in terms of accuracy and also makes available for study the participants' pauses and subvocal sounds. However, there may be situations in which tape recording might compromise the freedom with which the participant speaks, particularly if the interview covers sensitive areas and they have concerns about confidentiality. Some researchers (e.g. Orford, 1995) prefer to use hand-written accounts, which are felt to provide sufficient detail without leading to data overload.

ANALYSING AND DERIVING MEANING FROM TEXT

Usually, the quantitative approach asserts that data collection and data analysis should be discrete activities. However, in qualitative research this distinction is not made. Collection and analysis are inextricably bound together and inform each other in a reflexive manner to guide the development of a clear description of the data. After analysis has begun it is important to consider whether further data should be collected in order to provide more information on areas that are unclear.

The transcripts should be read over several times until the researcher is familiar with the material. Certainly at this stage it is very useful to have several people read them. This provides the opportunity to assess the reliability of the researcher's identification of topics in the data.

The major hurdle faced in qualitative analysis is the disparate, complex, and unstructured nature of the reams of transcription gathered. It is easy to baulk at this and either to retire from the research endeavour completely or to skim over a few pages and then form a general impression which is insufficient to do justice to the topic or the participants. A further risk is overestimating the significance of striking and vivid statements and dramatic events (Hopkinson *et al.*, 1995; Miles and Huberman, 1992) which are undoubtedly interesting to read but which do not really convey an accurate impression and depiction of the rest of the data.

The key to analysis is the development of a coding system. This allows a way into the mass of data. Codes provide a means of breaking down the data into categories which can then be investigated further. This can be done by gathering more data, often by asking questions directly about the categories or by exploring the categories in more detail. The researcher has to make a decision about how codes will be devised. It is possible to approach the data with a set of pre-existent coding categories which have been chosen on the basis of their appropriateness to the research question. For example, in an analysis of stress and coping, codes could be devised for references to stress-causing events and for coping strategies already expected by the researcher. The task, therefore, would be to identify references to these categories in the transcripts.

The alternative approach is to employ grounded theory (Glaser and Strauss, 1967) and to use the data itself to reveal the necessary codes. In this way, codes are developed from the references made in the data. Emergent theories which offer explanations and prompt further investigation begin to appear. Grounded theory is presented later in the chapter, with a research project offered as an example of how it can be used to present new theories.

On face value, this approach would seem to have an advantage in being less coercive. Certainly, it is possible to make data fit into already established, indeed expected, coding categories. However, it is arguable whether anyone can approach any data without some expectation of what they might find there. The formulation of a research question, the means by which data is elicited, and the beliefs possessed by the researcher all influence the way in which the data is interpreted. Given this, it is important to make these issues part of the research rather than to pretend that they do not matter. Declaring the position of the researcher on their chosen research topic is often undervalued. However, doing this is necessary if the inevitable allegations of impartiality are to be accounted for. As Starbuck and Nystrom (1984) put it, 'one can compensate for the biases one acknowledges, but not for the biases one denies'. Just as importantly, others can compensate for these admitted biases too.

Still on this subject, the beliefs and opinions of the researcher on qualitative research are worthy of consideration. Essentially, there are two schools of thought. On one hand are those who believe qualitative methods offer a better means of investigating all psychological issues than do quantitative methods. Often the holders of this view subscribe to the philosophy of social constructionism and challenge the notion of the 'subject' as passive and the researcher as an impartial observer. This view emphasizes the metaphorical nature of language.

Glachan (1996) makes the point that the researcher and the participants should have as much in common as possible in terms of ethnic background, gender, social class, and key life experiences. In this way misinterpretations and misunderstandings are less likely to occur. This viewpoint suggests that the role of the researcher is to make sense of the language used by the participants and to be sensitive to the meanings of their descriptions which may not be literal.

On the other hand are those who are essentially pragmatic about their choice of research methodologies and who use both qualitative and quantitative methods as research tools depending upon their appropriateness and not as articles of faith. Whilst this view does not necessarily reject the social mediation of the researcher/participant relationship, it tends to downplay this and concentrates on the practicalities of resolving the research problem.

Interpretation is ultimately an individual issue, influenced as it is by beliefs and concepts already held. For the reader of a qualitative research report, knowing the researcher's position on these areas assists in interpreting the conclusions they present. Thus the researcher should attempt to answer the following question: should the statements that participants make be taken literally as 'truthful' depictions of how they feel or should language use be considered as a socially constructed metaphor for communicating in a culturally appropriate manner?

The simplest criterion a code should meet is that it is easily understood by the researcher and effectively acts as shorthand for a more complex and varied set of phenomena referred to in the data. It is therefore useful to form the codes from a few letters of the main phenomena being described, e.g. 'HOM' to represent issues related to the home life of the participant. For the third interview presented earlier in this chapter, codes could be derived as follows:

HOMe: 'Actually, when I do take work home with me … I might as well have done it.'

LIAison: 'I'm always worried that when I do liaise it'll mean more work for me!'

At this stage the codes are quite loosely defined. The aim is to identify as broadly as possible the chief issues the participant is referring to so that further reading (and if necessary more data) may provide more detail.

After the initial codes have been identified, one should establish whether there are any areas that can be broken down into more detail and for which further sub-codes can be defined. The aim is a set of codes that effectively shadow the data, offering a means by which detail can be easily accessed. For example, the participant in the third interview makes a connection between worrying about work and the effect this has on her relationship with her husband. Both factors are considered to be negative in their effects. This can be illustrated in the coding system as follows:

HOM (−ve) ↔ RELationships (−ve) → unhappiness/stress

This indicates that worrying about work at home – 'I've spent all evening thinking about it' – leads to and is exacerbated by the effect it has on the husband – 'gets on my husband's nerves' – and this in turn is distressing.

Going further could reveal the following:

CONtrol (lack of) ↔ UNPredictability of work → DILatory behaviours

|
HOMe (−ve)

There is a connection between there never being enough time to do all the work that is necessary and behaviours that do not lead to work being completed, for example, 'I think, no, I'll call tomorrow.' However, this is exacerbated by issues such as unpredictability of workload and the feeling of lack of control this leads to. Indeed, this is the essence of stress. In this context, the 'dilatory' behaviours might actually be an ineffectual coping strategy, since they provide some short-term relief whilst ultimately conspiring to complete a very familiar vicious circle.

In this way, some initial codes will be found to be part of larger categories, others will be superseded by more appropriate interpretations of the evidence, and still others will be developed and found to be relatively independent and stable core concepts. In the example above, a core concept was the feelings of the participant about their lack of control over their work.

The use of codes is particularly useful for the comparison of statements made in multi-participant studies, where their conciseness and specificity can draw out similarities and identify differences.

Coding is an undeniably subjective process yet it offers considerable depth of analysis and understanding. If the coding is carried out independently by a number of researchers, then issues of inaccuracy and questionable interpretation can at least be identified. At all stages there remains the possibility of finding more data to check out problematic issues as they arise. Finally, when the remaining codes have been found to be suitably robust and accurate, conclusions can be drawn and illustrative examples used to support these.

AN EXAMPLE OF A RESEARCH PROJECT USING GROUNDED THEORY

A study of how registered mental nurses assess suicide risk for psychiatric in-patients used semi-structured interviews to collect data (Hardy, 1993). Despite the main aim being to identify current ward-based practices, what came out of the project was the psychological impact on the nurses of caring for suicidal patients. Using the grounded theory approach (Glaser and Strauss, 1967), an objective and rigorous study of the data was carried out. Categories were constructed alongside definitions, and new theories were drawn out of the natural and human conditions described (Melia, 1982; Hinds, 1984). Grounded theory is primarily an inductive approach to theory development. Despite this both inductive and deductive approaches were used to enable the researcher to develop theories on the research topic. Grounded theory also provides a structure upon which the researcher can think creatively (Field and Morse, 1992).

The approach to analysing the interviews was both inductive (constructing a theory that best helps to explain the observed relationship as it appears in the data) and deductive (constructs being derived from previous theory and tested against the evidence as it emerges from the data). Each individual interview was analysed for key words or phrases that emerged frequently or in patterns. Conclusions drawn from the data were formulated into an inducted theory for nursing the suicidal patient.

The effects of caring for a patient who either attempts or succeeds in suicide have received little previous research attention. Some of the nurses interviewed had personal experiences of friends or relatives who committed suicide as well as of patients they had cared for. The following quotations from the interviews descibe some of the emotions and frustrations encountered:

I had an experience of a patient I was primary nurse to [the allocated nurse responsible for the patient care throughout their treatment; Manthey, 1988] committing suicide. I remember thinking I'm glad she didn't do it whilst I was on duty and that was partly because I didn't want to take the blame and responsibility, and I realize that is a bit like just covering my back.

The other factor is that we've got a registration number and the fact that if a patient commits suicide on your ward there seems to be a swoop of admin- istrators and doctors all pointing the finger … that person can lose you your job'.

I've seen nurses leave after having to deal with a suicide and all the crap that goes with it. She was clinging on to his legs as he jumped and she couldn't save him, but there was still an inquest and she was hauled over the coals about it all.

I think the whole business of working with someone who is suicidal is very painful and it needs an awful lot of skill and insight and self-understanding. I think it's a rejection of you, isn't it, and all you have to offer. Ultimately you are the nurse, you have to be there all the time, and that's still not good enough. How can you offer help to someone when all they want is death?

From the data collected, words and phrases kept appearing that had strong emo- tional content. The nurses described feelings of anger, frustration, annoyance, dis- comfort, guilt, and blame. Staff stress levels were discussed and seen as associated with increased sickness rates at the time when a suicide was attempted or com- pleted on a ward. The nurses accounted for this as a way of coping and connected with having to control both their own emotions and the ward full of patients. 'People get fed up; nurses can detach themselves in an attempt to deal with all the stress.' One nurse described how the ward manager denied her the chance of going to a memorial service of a patient who had committed suicide by saying, 'We haven't got time for all that and besides sometimes it's worse to keep on about it.'

As a result of this project a revision was made to the guidelines on dealing with a suicide in hospital: they now recommend the provision of time and space for all patients and staff to contact the chaplaincy service – as a means of encouraging people to talk about the experience rather than avoid the topic. A staff counsellor has been appointed and a series of groups have developed which are looking at forming a staff support system throughout the hospital to offer debriefing and counselling (based on the Swindon staff support service, described in Chapter 10).

CONCLUSIONS

Qualitative methodologies offer much potential in occupational stress research. Since stress itself is a phenomenon that is based upon people's perceptions and feelings, there is a clear need to access these. Qualitative methods offer a means of making sense of what people say about stress and go a step beyond basic descriptions or entirely subjective, non-scientific opinions.

Nevertheless, qualitative methods do still lack the attraction of readily acceptable, scientific, quantitative methods and are open to accusations of bias. Since at present a qualitative approach is as much a frame of mind as a rigorous methodology, there is clearly a long way to go before the methods are fully unified and choices are made between them on a basis other than personal preference. Despite this, qualitative methods do offer a means for grappling with intangible, subjective experiences in an open and standardized manner. A method such as grounded theory at least makes the research and analysis process transparent.

Acknowledging and using the personal opinions and beliefs of both the researcher and the participant is a particularly powerful part of the qualitative approach. Aiming for a deeper understanding of the explanations and descriptions provided by participants, it offers a valuable alternative to the usual scientific concerns with generalizability. Qualitative methods could form a new paradigm for psychological enquiry and they certainly offer a valuable addition to quantitative approaches.

REFERENCES

Banister, P., Burman, E., Parker, I. *et al.* (1994) *Qualitative Methods in Psychology*, Open University Press, Buckingham.

Carson, J., Bartlett, H., Brown, B. and Hopkinson, P. (1995) Findings from the qualitative measures for CPNs, in *Stress and Coping in Mental Health Nursing* (eds J. Carson, L. Fagin, and S. Ritter), Chapman and Hall, London.

Field, D. and Morse, P. (1992) *Nursing Research. The Application of Qualitative Approaches*, Chapman and Hall, London.

Glachan, M. (1996) Balancing the qualitative and the quantitative in counselling psychology research. *Counselling Psychology Review*, **11** (1), 6–10.

Glaser, B.G. and Strauss, A.L. (1967) *The Discovery of Grounded Theory: Strategies for Qualitative Research*, Aldine, New York.

Good, D.A. and Watts, F.N. (1989) Qualitative research, in *Behavioural and Mental Health Research: A Handbook of Skills and Methods* (eds G. Parry and F.N. Watts), Lawrence Erlbaum Associates, Hove.

Green, A. (1995) Verbal protocol analysis. *The Psychologist*, March, 126–9.

Hardy, S.E. (1993) A quantitative study of how mental health nurses assess suicide risk. Dissertation. University of East London, Stratford. Unpublished.

Harper, D.J. (1994) The professional construction of paranoia and the discursive use of diagnostic criteria. *British Journal of Medical Psychology*, **67** (2), 131–43.

Henwood, K. and Pidgeon, P. (1992) Qualitative reseach and psychological theorising. *British Journal of Psychology*, **83**, 97–111.

Henwood, K. and Pidgeon, P. (1995) Grounded theory and psychological research. *The Psychologist*, March, 115–18.

Hinds, P.S. (1984) Inducing a definition of hope through the use of grounded theory methodology. *Journal of Advanced Nursing*, **9**, 357–62.

Hopkinson, P., Carson, J., Brown, D. *et al.* (1995) Stress in community mental health nursing: a qualitative study using focus groups. *Psychiatric Care*, **2** (3), 1–4.

Manthey, M. (1988) Myths that threaten. What primary nursing really is. *Nursing Management*, **19**, 54–6.

Melia, K.M. (1982) Tell it like it is – qualitative methodology and nursing research: understanding the student nurses' world. *Journal of Advanced Nursing*, **7**, 327–35.

Miles, M.B. and Huberman, A.M. (1992) *Qualitative Data Analysis – An Expanded Source Book*, 2nd edn, Sage Publications, London.

Orford, J. (1995) Qualitative research for applied psychologists. *Clinical Psychology Forum*, January, pp. 19–26.

Silverman, D. (1994) *Interpreting Qualitative Data – Methods for Analysing Talk, Text and Interaction*, Sage Publications, London.

Starbuck, W.H and Nystrom, P.C. (1984) Designing and understanding organisations, in *Handbook of Organisational Design* (eds W.H. Starbuck and P.C. Nystrom), Vol. 1, Oxford University Press, Oxford.

Wiseman, J. (1978) The research web, in *Social Research: Principles and Procedures* (eds J. Brynner and K. Stribley), Longman / Open University Press, London.

<table>
<tr><td>

15

</td><td>

Improving care by caring for professional carers

</td></tr>
</table>

Sally Hardy, Jerome Carson and Ben Thomas

In this concluding chapter we begin by reviewing some of the key issues emerging from the preceding chapters. We then consider the influential study on the Mental Health of the Workforce in NHS Trusts, the largest ever conducted in the British National Health Service, and probably also the largest worldwide. We describe one recently developed approach towards tackling stress at an organizational level. Finally, we summarize some of the key areas for future researchers and clinicians to address.

KEY ISSUES EMERGING FROM THIS BOOK

In Chapter 1, Kathleen Moore and Cary Cooper outline theories of stress. They present the 'stress as a stimulus model' and describe how it is measured. Then they focus on the 'stress as a response model' and how that is measured. Finally, they cover a range of 'interactional models' such as Holland's person–environment fit, psychobiological findings, Karasek's demand–discretion model, the cognitive model of Lazarus and Folkman, and lastly cybernetic models. They illustrate how the interactive components of stress, strain, environment, and personality can be measured using the Occupational Stress Indicator. This is undoubtedly the most sophisticated stress research tool yet developed, and, as they point out, is rapidly becoming the gold standard in occupational stress research. Moore and Cooper present stress models in an exceptionally lucid manner. Too much research in this area has not been grounded in stress theory, but has instead been based on *ad hoc* collections of questionnaires. The Occupational Stress Indicator is unique in combining theory with practical measurement of the stress process.

Sally Hardy and Ben Thomas summarize the literature on stress in health care professionals in Chapter 2. Although many articles are written about stress in the workplace, few emphasize the devastating effect it can have on the health care professional. This chapter looks specifically at nurses and medics and the connected phenomena of burnout and coping. By combining all the published literature, it can clearly be shown that the way an individual cognitively appraises a stressful situation, along with the level of support around them, can either help the professional carer cope and benefit from stress, or push them down the slippery slope of burnout and emotional exhaustion.

Chapter 3 focuses on the issue of stress in student health and social care professionals. Joe Tobin, Vedan Gunnoo and Jerome Carson present the findings of research they have conducted into stress among nursing and social work students. Unlike other groups of students, health and social care professionals experience both academic and clinical pressures. Both studies presented by these authors used relatively large samples. Caseness levels (as measured by a score of 5 or more on the General Health Questionnaire, GHQ-28) were twice as high for student social workers as for nursing students. Similarly, social work students had higher emotional exhaustion, depersonalization and burnout on the Maslach Scale. The authors conclude that social work students have significantly higher stress levels than have nursing students. However, they have as yet no explanation for this. Is it the case, for instance, that social work students are more neurotic as a group, hence are more prone to adverse stress reactions than are nursing students? Alternatively, is the process of training to be a social worker more stressful than training to be a nurse? Clearly, further research is needed to provide answers to these questions, probably utilizing longitudinal designs and qualitative methods.

In Chapter 4, Christopher Rance considers the interaction of organizational and intrapsychic perspectives, and how this relates to the experience of occupational stress. He draws from the work of Mead on the social origins of the personality, from psychoanalysis, and also from systems theory. Psychodynamic understandings have proved very important in developing our awareness of occupational stress. Issues such as boundaries, transference, and counter-transference are especially important in the field of mental health.

Sydney Brandon in Chapter 5 focuses on the health problems faced by doctors. He describes how doctors face unique difficulties in confronting their own health problems. He presents data on mortality rates, suicide, drug and alcohol consumption, and mental illness. He provides information on the National Counselling Service for Sick Doctors. He concludes that the expense and effort put into training doctors should be matched by a concern from the health service about their welfare.

Chapter 6 by Jerome Carson and Sally Hardy looks at the measurement of stress, coping, and occupational burnout syndrome in health care workers. They highlight the importance of adhering to strict psychometric principles, such as the reliability and validity of rating scales, in a field that is dominated by self-report measures. They also draw attention to factors such as absenteeism and turnover in assessing stress levels in organizations. Like Moore and Cooper, they also emphasize the importance of research being grounded in theory.

David Sines in Chapter 7 considers contextual factors and how we might enhance the competence of the work force. He describes how legislative changes in the British health and social care system have affected the work force. He raises the key issue that the success of any organization depends on the way it responds to the needs of its staff. He further argues that the work force needs to feel empowered, with access to decision making. However, he reflects that often this does not happen, and instead that rules are imposed on staff by managers. Given the huge organizational changes that the British health service is going through, Sines argues that to relieve stress in the workplace a range of mechanisms need to be in place to protect staff. These include opportunities for personal development, consistent feedback from managers to staff, freedom from threat, and the promise of job security. He concludes that careful attention to staff needs will lead to lower turnover, better standards of care, and an enhanced quality of life for patients.

In Chapter 8, Tony Butterworth describes the potential of clinical supervision as a tool for stress reduction in nursing, midwifery, and health visiting. He outlines how clinical supervision might be evaluated. He then summarizes the influential Clinical Supervision Evaluation Project, funded by the British Department of Health. This project is significant not least for the fact that it is spread across 23 research sites in two countries. He too finds much of value in the statement that 'happy nurse equals happy patient'.

Sally Hardy and her colleagues describe in Chapter 9 an in-patient unit for sick health care professionals. This chapter lays out the preliminary qualitative results of a study carried out at the first unit established solely for professional carers. The results of intensive interviews revealed common threads and a great sense of negative self-concept, which reinforces the stigma attached to mental health problems. All the professionals interviewed had strong ideas about how they should not behave. The sensitive information captured in the project merely reinforces the importance of continued work on occupational stress.

In Chapter 10, Jan Long tackles the issue of how support systems can be established to provide for the needs of health care staff. She reports on the Swindon staff support service, and notes that there are no groups of carers that do not require some form of support. The Swindon programme is uniquely for all grades of staff, from executive and administrative to clinical and ancillary staff. She identifies seven separate types of stress affecting health care workers: positive pressure; quantitative work overload; cumulative stress or compassion overload; post-traumatic stress; personal life crises; bullying and harassment at work; and combinations of the above. She then describes how the Swindon service tackles these various stressors. This service should serve as a model for other organizations concerned about the emotional welfare of their staff.

Mark Sutherland in Chapter 11 gives a personal perspective on staff support groups as a means of monitoring work stress. Drawing heavily on his own experiences of facilitating staff support groups, he illustrates the key elements that arise in such work, such as the process of providing interpretations.

Jerome Carson and Elizabeth Kuipers examine stress management interventions in Chapter 12. They illustrate how empirical research with different health and social care professionals can help elucidate the specific stressors that face particular groups of workers. Findings from these studies can then be used to feed into specific stress management interventions. They summarize a number of published studies, such as the impressive Louisville Medical School programme in the USA. They too emphasize the importance of theory–practice links. In concluding, they caution that however impressive stress management programmes may be, without concomitant organizational change they are unlikely to work in the long run.

In Chapter 13, Ben Thomas addresses the sensitive topic of staff selection. He discusses the importance of recruiting the right person for the job, both to meet the organization's needs and to ensure the person does not suffer unnecessary stress. Other stressful factors around recruitment are also considered, including discrimination and the selection process itself.

Finally, in Chapter 14, Patrick Hopkinson, Sally Hardy and Jerome Carson look at personal experiences of stress at work. The authors begin by presenting three accounts of work stress. They then outline a qualitative approach to studying work stress. They provide an example of a research project that utilizes grounded theory. They conclude that qualitative methods have much to offer in a field that is still largely dominated by quantitative approaches to stress.

MENTAL HEALTH OF THE WORK FORCE IN NHS TRUSTS

This influential study was conducted by the Institute of Work Psychology at the University of Sheffield and the Department of Psychology at the University of Leeds. The Phase 1 Final Report of this study was published in March 1996 (Borrill et al., 1996). This impressive study has four main research elements:

(1) A questionnaire survey.
(2) A psychiatric assessment study.
(3) A follow-up questionnaire survey.
(4) Intervention studies.

The researchers selected 20 health care trusts from among the 350 operating in England. Trusts were chosen from the eight health regions of England so as to be representative of the wider population of Trusts. Almost 12,000 staff participated in the study, a response rate of 50.5 per cent. Respondents were asked to complete a batch of questionnaires covering biographical information, work-related factors, and mental and physical health measures. Mental health was assessed using the 12 item version of the General Health Questionnaire. The average caseness rate on the GHQ-12 was 26.8 per cent for the total sample. Rates varied across different occupational groups. The most stressed group were managers (caseness rate = 33.4

per cent, $n = 925$), followed by nurses (= 28.5 per cent, $n = 4087$) and then doctors (= 27.8 per cent, $n = 1379$). The least stressed group were ancillary staff (= 20.1 per cent, $n = 740$). By linking their findings to other general population surveys that also used the GHQ-12, the researchers demonstrated that NHS staff have a higher caseness rate than the population at large. Interestingly the authors found higher caseness rates for female than for male managers (41 per cent versus 27 per cent), and for female than for male doctors (36 per cent versus 24 per cent). This trend was reversed for ancillary staff (17 per cent versus 24 per cent).

The sheer size and methodological rigour of this study means that it will be a landmark in the stress field. The findings reported above form only a small part of the total study. On account of its sample size it is unlikely ever to be replicated by other researchers. Despite this there are two main flaws in the study. Firstly, the measures selected do not reflect a coherent model of the stress process. If the researchers had chosen a measure like the Occupational Stress Indicator, this criticism could have been averted. Secondly, the lack of a qualitative focus to the study means that only partial explanations can be offered for some of the study's quantitative findings. For instance, the study as it stands cannot account for the difference in male and female doctor stress levels. Despite these minor criticisms, this study is destined to be one of the major studies in the stress field, if not the most important one ever conducted.

TACKLING STRESS AT WORK: AN ORGANIZATIONAL APPROACH

Two recent books produced by the British Health Education Authority on behalf of the National Health Service Executive describe organizational intervention to reduce work stress (Stapley et al., 1995; Stapley et al., 1996). Their approach is based on three key beliefs. Firstly, that work in the health services is by definition stressful. Secondly, the process of adapting to change (an organizational necessity in Britain's National Health Service) is inherently stressful. Thirdly, those who manage and work in the health service find themselves caught between society's infinite demand for health care and the reality of having only finite resources. The approach of Stapley and his colleagues draws heavily on the work of the Tavistock Institute in London. The influential research of Isabel Menzies Lyth (1988) suggests two critical principles for any stress management intervention:

- Health care staff are not solely victims of organizational stressors which impact on them from the outside. They may have an investment in and actually perpetuate some of the dysfunctional arrangements around them.
- Any process that aims to identify organizational sources of stress and tries to remedy them is likely to encounter unexpected resistance if the structures and procedures addressed have an unrecognised defensive function.

The model that these authors employ to tackle organizational stress is applied in five stages:

(1) *Initial action.* This involves meetings with the chief executive and senior staff. A 'stress management group' is formed to manage the programme. Data may be collected, such as sickness rates or expenditure on agency staff, to provide evidence of stress within the organization.

(2) *The listening group.* This is a two-day event for 25–30 people from different professions, functions, and levels within the organization. Led by external facilitators, the listening group aims to carry out a stress audit. It attempts to develop a preliminary analysis of the nature and extent of stress that might be affecting the Trust's performance.

(3) *Post listening group action.* The stress management group and the facilitator develop the format for the workshop that follows, to address the specific needs elicited. The group also selects the workshop participants.

(4) *Organizational stress workshop.* This is a second two-day event for 30–60 people attending as 'interest groups', led again by the external facilitators. This workshop aims to help participants develop their understanding of the dynamics in the organization that generate stress, and to apply that understanding to improve working relationships within the organization.

(5) *After the Workshop.* The stress management group manage and coordinate the dissemination and implementation of the workshop, with access to the external consultants.

This whole process is outlined in much greater detail by Stapley *et al.* (1996). In this second publication, the authors mention how they implemented their approach in three Trusts. However, they do not present information on the effectiveness of the programme. It would be interesting to conduct a systematic evaluative study looking at the comparative effectiveness of the organizational approach versus the individual approach across a range of health care settings. It may well be that neither approach is successful on its own, and that a combined model is best.

IMPROVING CARE BY CARING FOR PROFESSIONAL CARERS: KEY AREAS FOR RESEARCHERS AND CLINICIANS

Quis custodiet ipsos custodes? (Who guards the guards themselves?)

Some readers might ask why should we be concerned with the health of professional carers at all. If caring is a stressful business, and people are aware of this when they enter the professions, then why should they complain. Indeed some of the media make this very argument with respect to professional rescue workers, such as police officers and paramedics, who claim for compensation for post-traumatic stress disorder following involvement in major disasters (Black *et al.*, 1997). It is possible to make a number of counter arguments against such contentions. Firstly, few aspiring health and social care professionals are likely to really know in advance about the stresses that are likely to confront them in their chosen professions. Research into such stressors has emerged only in the last few years.

Secondly, it is the duty of all employers to look after the health of their work force. Thirdly, workers exposed to major trauma need our support not our condemnation. Employers need to develop debriefing procedures for staff involved in such disasters (Rosser, 1997). But who should guard the guards themselves?

In Chapter 12, Carson and Kuipers argued the need for greater collaboration between occupational or organizational specialists and clinical workers. The large study on the Mental Health of the Workforce in NHS Trusts (Borrill *et al.*, 1996), described earlier, is an example of just such a collaboration. Such work is, however, expensive to carry out. There is an onus on professional bodies to sponsor such work. For instance the English National Board, which oversees all nursing, midwifery, and health visitor education, might sponsor research into investigating and alleviating stress in student nurses. Equally, while the Government has sponsored some research into the health of the NHS work force, more work in this area is clearly needed. Definitive research studies are very difficult to mount and have a frustrating tendency not to have clear-cut conclusions. What sort of studies do we therefore need?

Two major types of study are required. Firstly, investigative studies. Secondly, interventions. The vast majority of research to date has been cross-sectional in nature. That is, health and social care professionals are assessed on only one occasion, and conclusions drawn from that single data point. We therefore know little about the natural history of conditions such as occupational burnout syndrome. Analysis of data collected by some of our own research team (Fagin *et al.*, 1996) suggests that a mere 33 out of 648 (5 per cent) of ward-based mental health nurses could be described as suffering from occupational burnout syndrome. To find 100 nurses suffering from this syndrome would therefore require us to sample some 2000 nurses. We need to follow up such nurses to see what happens to them. Do they end up leaving the profession, or do they stay and have a negative influence on their co-workers? Equally, we might focus on staff who clearly do not suffer from burnout or who seem to be burnout resistant. We have calculated that some 66 of our 648 (10 per cent) mental health nurses fall into this category. What can we learn from burnout resistant staff? It is likely that future research will focus more on developing resilience in staff, in the same way that resilience is now being studied in the spouses of the mentally ill (Mannion, 1996). Such work really falls into the domain of qualitative research. Having identified 'vulnerable' and potentially 'invulnerable' staff, probably by using quantitative methods, we then need to go back and conduct individual interviews and focus groups to develop a better understanding of burnout. This knowledge can then help us to develop more effective intervention strategies.

It seems likely that future intervention strategies will need to incorporate organizational aspects as well as clinical stress management training. There may be certain aspects of clinical environments that are bound to cause stress to most staff exposed to them. Accident and emergency departments on Friday and Saturday evenings especially can be very stressful places to work, with some patients arriving in an intoxicated and aggressive state. Such patients are likely to cause all staff stress, irrespective of their coping or resilience skills. An organizational intervention that might reduce staff stress in such situations might be to employ security staff, who could provide immediate assistance in the event of any staff member being assaulted. Employers need to ask the question: what can they do to minimize the stress under which staff are expected to deliver a clinical service? Health and social care organizations are, however, complex systems with many different staff groupings. What stresses particular groups of staff? While we have developed measures of stress in mental health nurses, such measures will have very limited application with other groups such as ancillary or secretarial staff. There is a need therefore to utilize measures such as Cooper's Occupational Stress Indicator which can be applied to all groups of staff. Rees and Smith (1991) did this for one large health care provider, and were able to present one of the first stress league tables. Health and social care professionals need to conduct stress audits of their staff to identify what aspects of the work environment the staff find most stressful. They then need to consider what organizational changes could be made to reduce stress.

Clinically based interventions are likely to be multimodal in nature. It is highly unlikely that one method of stress reduction, such as relaxation training, will benefit all staff (Kolbell, 1995). Rather it is important to identify specific areas that individuals may need to build up to develop their stress tolerance. Elsewhere (see Chapter 12) we have described such stress tolerance factors as 'mediating or buffering' factors. They are likely to include the individual's sense of self-esteem, the presence or absence of social support, hardiness or resilience, coping skills, a sense of mastery or personal control, emotional stability, and having good physiological release mechanisms. To be maximally effective, interventions need to be targeted on only those areas where an individual may have difficulty. For instance staff scoring below cut-off points on self-esteem scales such as the Rosenberg Trait and Heatherton State Scales might benefit from some guidance on self-esteem enhancement. However, we would not need to offer such training to staff already scoring high on self-esteem. Staff stress interventions are highly complex and require careful design (Martin, 1992). The sheer variety and range of the interventions on offer is well illustrated in books by Quick, Murphy and Hurrell (1992), and Murphy *et al.* (1995).

In the development of work-based interventions it is critical that interventions be properly scientifically evaluated and not based on the latest fads. Again we would emphasize that evaluation requires the combined skills of occupational and clinical specialists. Thomas (1996) has summarized many of the key principles of such evaluation, which are likely to become even more important in an era of evidence-based medicine (Sackett *et al.*, 1996).

In our opinion, we can improve standards of patient care by attending to the needs of professional carers. As has been emphasized several times in this book, 'happy nurse equals happy patient'. We all have an obligation to ensure that staff needs are provided for, as well as patient needs. Health and social care services that do not look after the needs of their staff are not just failing their staff – ultimately they may be failing their patients.

REFERENCES

Black, D., Newman, M., Harris-Hendriks, J. and Mezey, G. (eds) (1997) *Psychological Trauma: A Developmental Approach*, Gaskell, London.

Borrill, C.,Wall, T., West, M. *et al.* (1996) *Mental Health of the Workforce in NHS Trusts.* Institute of Work Psychology, University of Sheffield.

Fagin, L., Carson, J., Leary, J. *et al.* (1996) Stress, coping and burnout in mental health nurses: findings from three research studies. *The International Journal of Social Psychiatry*, **42** (2), 102–11.

Kolbell, R. (1995) When relaxation is not enough, in *Job Stress Interventions* (eds L. Murphy, J. Hurrell, S. Sauter and G. Puryear Keita), American Psychological Association, Washington.

Mannion, E. (1996) Resilience and burden in spouses of people with mental illness. *Psychiatric Rehabilitation Journal*, **20** (2), 13–23.

Martin, E. (1992) Designing stress training, in *Stress and Well-Being at Work: Assessments and Interventions for Occupational Mental Health* (eds J. Quick, L. Murphy. and J. Hurrell), American Psychological Association, Washington.

Menzies Lyth, I. (1988) *Containing Anxiety in Institutions: Selected Essays*. Vol. 1, Free Association Books, London.

Murphy, L., Hurrell, J., Sauter, S. and Puryear Keita, G. (eds) (1995) *Job Stress Interventions*. American Psychological Association, Washington.

Quick, J., Murphy, L. and Hurrell, J. (eds) (1992) *Stress and Well-Being at Work: Assessments and Interventions for Occupational Mental Health*, American Psychological Association, Washington.

Rees, D. and Smith, S. (1991) Work stress in occupational therapists assessed by the Occupational Stress Indicator. *British Journal of Occupational Therapy*, **54** (8), 289–94.

Rosser, R. (1997) Effects of disasters on helpers, in *Psychological Trauma: A Developmental Approach* (eds D. Black, M. Newman, J. Harris-Hendriks and G. Mezey), Gaskell, London.

Sackett, D., Rosenberg, W., Gray, J. *et al.* (1996) Evidence based medicine: what it is and what it isn't. *British Medical Journal*, **312**, 71–2.

Stapley, L., Cleavely, E., Dartington, T. *et al.* (1995) *Organisational Stress in the National Health Service*, Health Education Authority, London.

Stapley, L., Cardona, F., Cleavely, E. *et al.* (1996) *Organisational Stress: Planning and Implementing a Programme to Address Organisational Stress in the NHS*, Health Education Authority, London.

Thomas, B. (1996) Principles of evaluation, in *Collaborative Community Mental Health Care* (eds M. Watkins, N. Hervey, J. Carson and S. Ritter), Edward Arnold, London.

Index

Page numbers in **bold** refer to figures and page numbers in *italic* refer to tables.